Finding your balance , a guide to stability in life

BALANCE ISSUE, Volume 1

George

Published by George, 2024.

FINDING YOUR BALANCE , A GUIDE TO STABILITY IN LIFE

First edition. October 14, 2024.

Copyright © 2024 George.

ISBN: 979-8227649089

Written by George.

Table of Contents

Chapter 1

Finding Your Balance: A Guide to Stability in Life

The problem of "Unsteadiness or Loss of Balance" in various aspects of life where individuals or communities experience instability is common . This could relate to mental health issues, physical challenges like balance, social dynamics, or even environmental concerns. The book aims to provide insights into recognizing signs of unsteadiness, understanding underlying causes, and offering practical strategies to regain balance. It may also include personal stories, expert interviews, and actionable steps for readers to achieve a more stable life.

How balance is maintained

Balance is maintained through a complex interplay of sensory systems, neural processing, and muscular responses. Here's a breakdown of how balance is achieved:

Key Systems Involved in Maintaining Balancc

1. Sensory Input

Three primary systems provide crucial information to the brain about the body's position and movement:

- **Vestibular System**: Located in the inner ear, this system detects motion and changes in head position. It helps sense linear movements (like moving up and down) and rotational movements (like turning your head). The vestibular organs send signals to the brain about your orientation relative to gravity.

- **Visual System**: The eyes provide visual cues about the environment, helping to maintain orientation. They help determine where you are in space and can compensate for any imbalance by providing a frame of reference.
- **Proprioceptive System**: This consists of sensory receptors located in muscles and joints that provide information about body position and movement. It helps the brain understand where different body parts are located without looking at them.

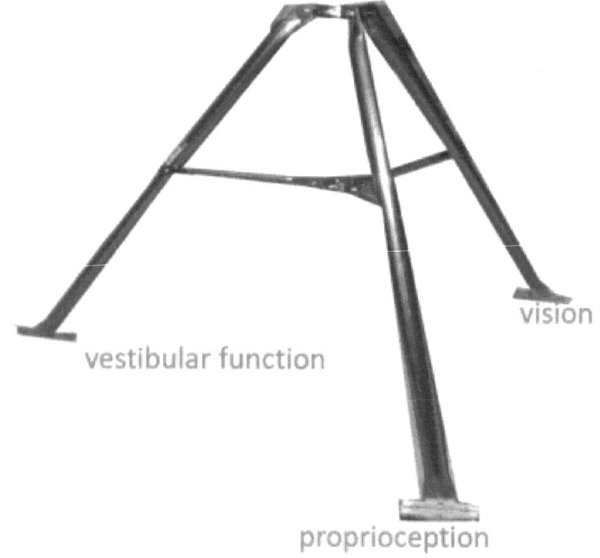

. **Types of Balance**

Balance can be categorized into two main types:

- **Static Balance**: This refers to maintaining equilibrium while stationary, such as standing still.

. **Dynamic Balance**: This involves maintaining stability while in motion, such as walking or running.

Conclusion

In summary, balance is maintained through a sophisticated network involving sensory input from the vestibular, visual, and proprioceptive systems, central processing in the brain, and coordinated motor output to muscles. This integrated approach allows individuals to stay upright and navigate their environment effectively, adapting quickly to changes or disturbances.

Balance disorders can affect individuals of all ages, and understanding who experiences these disorders and why they matter is crucial for addressing their impact on daily life.

2. Central Processing

The brain integrates information from these three systems to maintain balance. The central nervous system (CNS) processes sensory input, particularly from the vestibular system, visual system, and proprioceptors, to create a cohesive understanding of body position and movement.

. **Cerebellum**: This part of the brain plays a critical role in coordinating balance and movement. It receives input from all three sensory systems and helps adjust muscle activity to maintain stability.
. **Brainstem**: The brainstem processes balance-related information and sends signals to the muscles that

control posture and movement.

3. Motor Output

Once the brain has processed the sensory information, it generates appropriate motor responses to maintain balance:

- **Muscle Activation**: The brain sends signals to various muscles throughout the body to contract or relax as needed, helping to keep the center of mass over the base of support (the area beneath your feet).
- **Postural Adjustments**: When there is a disturbance (like tripping or being pushed), the body automatically makes adjustments through reflexes that involve rapid muscle contractions to regain balance.

Understanding Balance Disorders

Loss of balance refers to a condition where a person feels unsteady or has difficulty in maintaining their equilibrium while standing or walking or even sitting. This can lead to feelings of dizziness or vertigo, where the individual may perceive that they or their surroundings are spinning or they can't fix the eyes on objects.

Key Points About Loss of Balance

Causes: Loss of balance can arise from various factors, including:

- **Inner ear problems**: The inner ear plays a crucial

role in maintaining balance. Conditions like infections or other disorders (e.g., Meniere's disease) can disrupt this function.

- **Neurological issues**: Conditions such as strokes, multiple sclerosis, or Parkinson's disease or tumor can affect the brain's ability to process balance-related information.
- **Medications**: Some medications can cause dizziness or affect coordination, leading to balance issues.
- **Aging**: As people age, changes in the body can increase the risk of balance problems.
- **Cardiac conditions ;** causing insufficient perfusion of blood into brain
- **Medical** causes like anemia
- **Ophthalmologic** conditions like poor vision
- **Orthopedic conditions** causing loss of ability to maintain the center of gravity of body
- **psychiatric** conditions rarely can cause unsteadiness

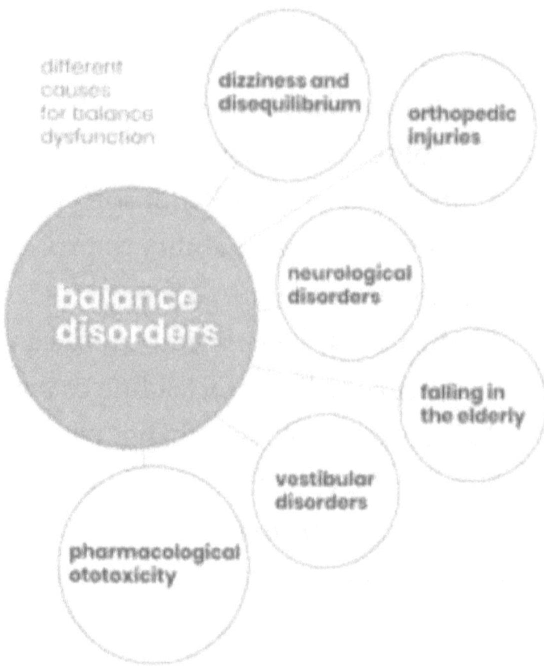

Symptoms: Common symptoms associated with loss of balance include:

- Dizziness or lightheadedness
- A feeling of spinning (vertigo)
- Staggering when trying to walk
- Increased risk of falls
- As if falling to oneside or feeling of falling from a height,or feeling of travelling in a boat in the sea, or seesaw movements, rocking in a chair

Impact: Balance problems can significantly affect daily life, making it challenging to perform routine activities and increasing the risk of injuries from falls.

If someone experiences persistent loss of balance, it is advisable to consult a healthcare professional for evaluation and potential treatment options.

What are the most common causes of balance issues ?

Loss of balance can be caused by a variety of factors, often related to issues with the inner ear, neurological conditions, medications, or physical injuries. Here are some of the most common causes of balance issues:

1. Inner Ear Problems

Benign Paroxysmal Positional Vertigo (BPPV): This is the leading cause of vertigo, triggered by changes in head position. It occurs when tiny calcium crystals in the inner ear become dislodged, leading to brief episodes of intense spinning sensations. It is estimated that BPPV affects about **10 to 64 per 100,000 people per year**. The incidents are given in the table

Metric	Percentage/Rate
Lifetime Prevalence	2.4%
1-Year Prevalence	1.6%
Annual Incidence	0.6% (64 per 100,000)
Cumulative Incidence (age 80)	~10%
Gender Ratio (Women:Men)	3.2% : 1.6%

- The inner ear contains structures crucial for maintaining balance. Conditions such as labyrinthitis (inflammation of the inner ear) and Meniere's disease (which affects fluid balance in the ear) can lead to dizziness and imbalance

2. Neurological Conditions

Disorders that affect the brain and nervous system, such as **multiple sclerosis, Parkinson's**

disease, and **strokes**, can disrupt the body's ability to maintain balance. These conditions may impair coordination and lead to unsteadiness

Migraine-associated vertigo, commonly referred to as vestibular migraine, can cause vertigo in a significant number of individuals who experience migraines. This condition is characterized by episodes of dizziness or vertigo that may occur with or without accompanying headache symptoms.

Frequency and Characteristics of Vertigo in Migraine Patients

Prevalence of Vertigo in Migraine

Research indicates that up to **25% of patients with migraines** experience vertigo as a symptom

. Additionally, studies suggest that more than **50% of migraine sufferers** report some form of balance disorder, making migraine-related vertigo one of the most common causes of spontaneous episodic vertigo

3. **Medications**

Certain medications can have side effects that impact balance. Common culprits include **antidepressants**, **antihistamines**, **sleeping pills**, and medications for anxiety or high blood pressure. These can cause dizziness or sedation, increasing the risk of falls

4. Physical Injuries

Injuries, particularly those affecting the head or limbs, can lead to balance problems. For instance, a concussion can disrupt normal balance function, while broken bones or muscle injuries may hinder movement coordination

5. Aging

As people age, changes in the body can contribute to balance issues. Factors such as decreased muscle strength, joint problems (like arthritis), and sensory decline (vision and proprioception) increase the likelihood of experiencing balance difficulties

6. Vision Problems

Impaired vision from conditions like cataracts or macular degeneration can affect spatial awareness and balance. The eyes play a critical role in helping maintain equilibrium by providing visual cues about surroundings

7.cervical vertigo

also known as cervicogenic dizziness, is a type of dizziness that arises from issues related to the cervical spine (neck). This condition is characterized by a sensation of spinning or disorientation, often accompanied by neck pain. It typically occurs after specific neck movements or postures and can significantly impact balance and coordination

Cervical vertigo can stem from various factors, including:

- **Neck Injuries**: Trauma such as whiplash from car accidents can disrupt normal neck function and lead to dizzines

Poor Posture: Prolonged poor neck posture may contribute to the development of cervical vertigo

Arterial Issues: Conditions like atherosclerosis or arterial dissection can block blood flow to the inner ear or brainstem, causing dizziness

Degenerative Conditions: Osteoarthritis and cervical spondylosis can affect the cervical spine's structure and function

Muscle Spasms: Tension in neck muscles can also play a role in triggering symptoms

8. Circulatory Issues

Problems with blood circulation, such as low blood pressure (orthostatic hypotension), can cause dizziness when standing up quickly, leading to balance problems

9. Sedentary Lifestyle

A lack of physical activity can weaken muscles and reduce coordination, making it harder to maintain balance, especially in older adults

Understanding these causes is crucial for addressing balance issues effectively, as treatment may vary depending on the underlying condition contributing to the problem. If someone experiences persistent balance difficulties, consulting a healthcare professional is recommended for proper diagnosis and management.

what are the different types of balance loss symptoms
Loss of balance can manifest through various symptoms, which often indicate underlying issues with the vestibular system, neurological health, or other bodily functions. Here are the most common symptoms associated with balance disorders:

Common Symptoms of Balance Loss

1. **Dizziness or Vertigo**

- A spinning sensation or feeling lightheaded, even when stationary. This is often described as a feeling that you or your surroundings are moving.

2. **Unsteadiness**
   - Difficulty maintaining stability while standing or walking, leading to a feeling of being off-balance.

3. **Falling or Fear of Falling**
   - Experiencing actual falls or a persistent fear of falling can significantly affect daily activities and confidence.

4. **Staggering**
   - Walking in an unsteady manner, similar to being intoxicated, which can occur when trying to move.

5. **Lightheadedness**
   - A sensation of faintness or feeling as if you might pass out, often accompanied by a floating feeling.

6. **Blurred Vision**
   - Difficulty focusing or seeing clearly, which can contribute to balance problems as vision is crucial for maintaining equilibrium.

7. **Disorientation or Confusion**
   - Feeling disoriented in space or having trouble understanding where you are, which can lead to difficulty in navigating environments.

8. **Sensitivity to Motion**
   - Increased sensitivity to movement, such as feeling dizzy when turning your head quickly

or when in a moving vehicle.

9. **Nausea and Vomiting**
   - These symptoms can accompany dizziness and are particularly common in cases of severe vertigo.

10. **Changes in Heart Rate and Blood Pressure**
    - Fluctuations in these vital signs may occur alongside balance issues, especially when standing up quickly (orthostatic hypotension).

11. **Anxiety or Panic**
    - Feelings of anxiety may arise due to the unpredictability of balance loss, leading to avoidance behaviors.

Conclusion

These symptoms can vary in intensity and duration, and they may come and go over time. If someone experiences persistent balance issues, it's important to consult a healthcare professional for proper evaluation and treatment options tailored to the underlying causes of their symptoms

Overview of Who Experiences Balance Disorders

1. Children and Teens

- **Symptoms**: Kids and teens may appear clumsy or uncoordinated, struggling with activities like walking, riding a bike, or participating in sports. They might experience dizziness, lightheadedness, or disorientation but may not always be able to articulate their feelings

Causes: Balance issues in younger populations can arise from ear infections, head injuries, vestibular disorders, or even genetic predispositions to conditions like migraines

2. **Adults**

Prevalence: Approximately 15% of American adults experience balance or dizziness problems at some point

These issues can stem from various health conditions, medications, or inner ear problems.

Symptoms: Adults may experience dizziness, vertigo, unsteadiness, and difficulty concentrating

3. **Elderly**

. **High Risk**: Balance disorders are particularly common among older adults. About 19.6% of elderly individuals report experiencing balance problems annually

Impact: The elderly are more prone to falls due to weakened muscles, joint issues, and other health conditions that affect balance. This demographic often faces significant repercussions from falls, including serious injuries like fractures

Why Balance Disorders Matter

1. **Impact on Daily Life**

- Balance disorders can profoundly affect an individual's ability to perform everyday activities. For children, this might mean difficulties in school or sports; for adults and the elderly, it can hinder mobility and independence

2. Psychological Effects

- The fear of falling or experiencing dizziness can lead to anxiety and social withdrawal. This is particularly relevant for the elderly, who may limit their activities due to concerns about losing balance

3. Increased Risk of Injury

- Individuals with balance disorders are at a higher risk of falls and related injuries. Falls are a leading cause of injury among older adults and can result in long-term disability or even death

4. Need for Treatment and Rehabilitation

- Understanding balance disorders is essential for effective treatment. Many cases require physical therapy or vestibular rehabilitation to improve balance and reduce symptoms. Early intervention can help mitigate the effects of balance disorders on quality of life

In summary, balance disorders can affect a wide range of individuals—from children to the elderly—impacting their physical health and emotional well-being. Recognizing the significance of these disorders is vital for facilitating appropriate care and improving overall quality of life.

Chapter 2: The Science Behind Balance

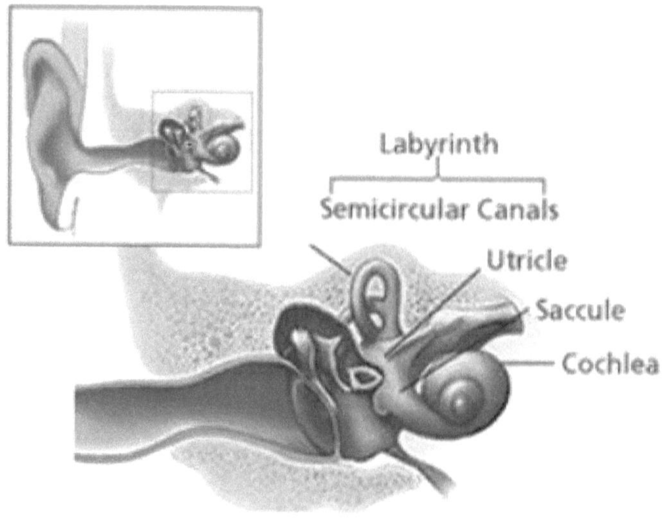

- Introduction to the vestibular system and its role.

The vestibular system is a crucial component of the inner ear responsible for maintaining balance and spatial orientation. It detects head movements and position relative to gravity, enabling the body to respond appropriately to maintain stability.

Overview of the Vestibular System

The vestibular system is primarily located in the **inner ear**, consisting of two main structures: the **semicircular canals** and the **otolith organs** (utricle and saccule).

- **Semicircular Canals**: These three canals are oriented at right angles to each other and are sensitive to rotational movements. Each canal is filled with fluid (endolymph) and contains sensory cells that detect changes in head rotation.
- **Otolith Organs**: The utricle and saccule detect linear accelerations and gravitational forces. They contain hair cells embedded in a gelatinous layer topped with tiny calcium carbonate crystals (otoconia), which shift with movement, stimulating the hair cells

Functions of the Vestibular System
The vestibular system serves several key functions:

- **Balance Maintenance**: By providing information about head position and movement, the vestibular system helps maintain an upright posture. This is achieved through reflexes that adjust muscle tone and posture based on sensory input from the vestibular apparatus

- **Spatial Orientation**: The system allows individuals to perceive their orientation in three-dimensional space, facilitating coordinated movements. This is essential for activities such as walking, running, or any dynamic motion where balance is critical

Gaze Stabilization: The vestibulo-ocular reflex (VOR) is a critical mechanism that stabilizes vision during head movements by coordinating eye movements in the opposite direction of head motion, ensuring that visual images remain clear

Mechanisms of Action

1. **Detection of Movement**:
   - The semicircular canals respond to angular acceleration. When the head rotates, fluid movement within these canals bends hair cells, generating nerve impulses that inform the brain about the direction and speed of rotation.
   - The otolith organs respond to linear acceleration and tilt. Changes in position cause otoconia to shift, bending hair cells and sending signals regarding head orientation relative to gravity
2. **Neural Pathways**:
   - Signals from the vestibular organs travel via the vestibulocochlear nerve (cranial nerve VIII) to various brain regions, including the cerebellum, brainstem, and thalamus. These areas process vestibular information and coordinate appropriate motor responses for balance and posture
3. **Reflex Actions**:

- ○ The vestibulospinal reflex (VSR) helps stabilize posture by adjusting muscle activity in response to changes detected by the vestibular system. For instance, if a person is pushed, this reflex activates muscles to counteract the force and maintain balanceConclusion

In summary, the vestibular system plays an integral role in maintaining balance and spatial orientation through its detection of head movements and position. By integrating sensory information from both internal structures and external cues, it enables rapid adjustments that keep an individual stable during various activities. Understanding its functions is essential for diagnosing balance disorders and developing effective rehabilitation strategies.

How does the vestibular system interact with vision and proprioception

The connection between the inner ear, eyes, and brain in maintenance of balance

The connection between the inner ear, eyes, and brain is vital for maintaining balance and spatial orientation. This intricate relationship primarily involves the vestibular system, which integrates sensory information from the inner ear with visual input and proprioceptive feedback from the body.

Components of the Balance System

Inner Ear

The **inner ear** contains the vestibular apparatus, which includes:

- **Semicircular Canals**: These detect rotational movements of the head. Each canal is oriented at right angles to the others, enabling the detection of motion in three-dimensional space.
- **Otolith Organs**: Comprising the utricle and saccule, these organs sense linear accelerations and gravitational forces.

Eyes

The **eyes** play a crucial role through the **vestibulo-ocular reflex (VOR)**. This reflex stabilizes vision by coordinating eye movements with head movements. When the head turns, the VOR ensures that the eyes move in the opposite direction, keeping the visual field steady.

Brain

The **brain** processes information from both the vestibular system and visual inputs to maintain balance. Key areas involved include:

- **Vestibular Nuclei**: Located in the brainstem, these nuclei integrate signals from the vestibular system and send outputs to control eye movements and posture.
- **Cerebellum**: This region fine-tunes motor responses based on input from both vestibular and visual systems, helping to adjust balance and coordination.

Mechanisms of Coordination

1. **Sensory Integration**:

- The vestibular system detects head position and movement through hair cells in the semicircular canals and otolith organs. These cells send signals via the vestibulocochlear nerve (CN VIII) to the brainstem

Visual information from the eyes is processed to determine orientation and movement relative to external objects

1. **Reflex Actions**:
   - The VOR is a critical reflex that adjusts eye movements based on head motion. For example, when turning the head to the right, signals from the left semicircular canal stimulate eye muscles to move the eyes leftward, maintaining focus on a target
   - The vestibulospinal reflex (VSR) stabilizes posture by adjusting muscle tone throughout the body in response to changes detected by the vestibular system
2. **Feedback Loops**:
   - The cerebellum continually compares inputs from both sensory systems (vestibular and visual) to ensure coordinated responses. If discrepancies arise—such as when visual inputs suggest no movement while vestibular inputs indicate motion—this can lead to conditions like motion sickness

Conclusion

In summary, maintaining balance involves a complex interplay between the inner ear, eyes, and brain. The vestibular system provides essential information about head position and movement, while visual input helps orient this information within a broader spatial context. Together, these systems enable precise coordination of eye movements and body posture, ensuring stability during various activities.

What are the Factors that can disrupt balance (e.g., aging, injuries, medical conditions ?

Several factors can disrupt balance, affecting individuals across different age groups and health conditions. Understanding these factors is essential for developing effective prevention and intervention strategies.

Key Factors Disrupting Balance

1. Aging

As individuals age, physiological changes can impair balance. This includes deterioration in vision, vestibular function, and proprioception (the sense of body position). Older adults often experience decreased muscle strength and flexibility, further contributing to balance issues

2. Injuries

Injuries, particularly to the lower extremities or spine, can significantly impact balance. Fractures, sprains, or surgeries may lead to reduced mobility and strength, making it difficult for individuals to maintain stability during movement

3. Medical Conditions

Various medical conditions can disrupt balance:

- **Neurological Disorders**: Conditions such as Parkinson's disease, multiple sclerosis, and stroke can affect the central nervous system, leading to coordination problems and balance impairments
- **Vestibular Disorders**: Inner ear issues like vertigo or vestibular neuritis can cause dizziness and a false sense of motion, severely impacting balance
- **Diabetic Neuropathy**: This condition affects peripheral nerves, leading to reduced sensation in the feet and legs, which can hinder balance

4. Medications

Certain medications can have side effects that impair balance. Common culprits include antihypertensives (which may cause dizziness) and sedatives. It's crucial for individuals to discuss potential side effects with healthcare providers

5. Strength and Endurance

Weakness in core and leg muscles can limit an individual's ability to make necessary adjustments to maintain balance. Poor muscle endurance may lead to fatigue during activities, increasing the risk of falls

6. Pain

Chronic pain conditions can limit mobility and strength, making it difficult for individuals to engage in activities that support balance. Pain in areas like the back or knees often leads to compensatory movements that can further destabilize an individual

7. Vision Impairments

Vision plays a critical role in maintaining balance by providing spatial awareness. Conditions such as cataracts or macular degeneration can impair visual input, making it challenging to navigate environments safely

8. Environmental Factors

External conditions like uneven surfaces, poor lighting, or slippery floors can pose significant challenges to maintaining balance. Awareness of these factors is essential for fall prevention strategies

Conclusion

Balance is influenced by a complex interplay of physical capabilities, medical conditions, environmental factors, and sensory inputs. Addressing these factors through targeted interventions—such as strength training, vision correction, pain management, and environmental modifications—can significantly enhance stability and reduce the risk of falls.

Simple illustrations and analogies to explain complex concepts

To explain the complex concepts of balance maintenance, simple illustrations and analogies can be highly effective. Here are several metaphors that capture the essence of maintaining balance in various contexts:

FINDING YOUR BALANCE , A GUIDE TO STABILITY IN LIFE

Illustrations and Analogies for Balance

1. Riding a Bicycle

Albert Einstein famously stated, "Life is like riding a bicycle. To keep your balance, you must keep moving." This analogy highlights that just as a cyclist must continuously pedal to maintain stability, individuals must keep progressing through life's challenges to maintain their equilibrium. Stopping or hesitating can lead to losing balance, emphasizing the importance of adaptability and ongoing effort in life

2. Tightrope Walking

Balancing on a tightrope requires focus, precision, and constant adjustments. This metaphor illustrates how maintaining balance in life—whether between work and personal commitments or emotional stability—demands similar skills. One misstep can lead to a fall, but with practice and determination, one can learn to navigate these challenges gracefully

3. Seesaw Dynamics

A seesaw represents the need for constant adjustment in balancing different aspects of life. Unlike a static scale that seeks equal weight on both sides, a seesaw acknowledges movement and interaction. When one side is heavier, adjustments must be made to regain balance. This metaphor encourages individuals to recognize when they are off-balance and make necessary tweaks to restore equilibrium

4. Baking a Muffin

The process of baking a muffin at different temperatures serves as an analogy for balance in life. Baking at 1,000 degrees for three minutes results in a charred muffin, while baking at 325 degrees for fifteen minutes yields a perfectly cooked treat. This metaphor illustrates that achieving balance often requires patience and moderation rather than rushing through tasks or experiences

5. Dancing

Dance requires rhythm and coordination, much like maintaining balance in life. Each step must be executed with care and awareness of one's surroundings. Just as dancers adjust their movements based on the music and partners, individuals must adapt their actions based on changing circumstances to maintain harmony and stability

6. Tree Roots

A tree's roots provide stability against strong winds and storms, symbolizing how personal values and beliefs can ground individuals during turbulent times. Just as roots anchor a tree, having a strong foundation in one's principles helps maintain balance amid life's challenges

7. Sunlight Distribution

The sun distributes its light evenly across the Earth, which can be likened to the need for an even distribution of energy and attention among various life aspects—work, family, and personal time. Striving for this balanced allocation helps prevent burnout and ensures that each area receives the attention it deserves

Conclusion

These metaphors effectively illustrate the complex concepts of maintaining balance by drawing parallels with familiar experiences. Whether through the dynamic nature of riding a bicycle or the careful adjustments required in tightrope walking, these analogies emphasize that achieving balance involves continuous effort, adaptability, and mindfulness.

Chapter 3: Recognizing Your Own Imbalances

Self-assessment tools for identifying balance issues are essential for individuals, especially older adults, to gauge their stability and risk of falls. Here's a summary of some widely recognized tools:

1. Activities-Specific Balance Confidence Scale (ABC)

- **Description**: This is a 16-item questionnaire where respondents rate their confidence in maintaining balance during various daily activities.
- **Scoring**: Each item is rated from 0% (no confidence) to 100% (complete confidence), with the average score indicating overall confidence.
- **Advantages**:
    - Relates directly to daily activities.
    - Quick to administer (about 15 minutes).
    - Good test-retest reliability (ICC ranging from 0.7 to 0.92).
- **Limitations**: It is subjective and does not identify specific types of balance problems or relate directly to fall risk

2. Balance Evaluation Systems Test (BESTest)

- **Description**: A comprehensive tool that assesses multiple systems affecting balance through 36 items divided into six categories, including biomechanical constraints and sensory orientation.
- **Scoring**: Each item is scored on a scale from 0 (worst performance) to 3 (best performance), with total scores

expressed as a percentage of the maximum possible score.

- **Advantages**:
    - Identifies specific balance deficits.
    - Guides targeted interventions based on identified issues.
    - High inter-rater reliability (ICC = 0.91).
- **Limitations**: Time-consuming (approximately 35 minutes) and requires various equipment

3. Four Stage Balance Test

- **Description**: This test evaluates static balance through four progressively challenging standing positions, such as standing on one foot and tandem stance.
- **Method**: Participants are timed on how long they can maintain each position without support.
- **Outcome**: Inability to hold the tandem stance for at least 10 seconds indicates an increased risk of falls.
- **Reliability**: Moderate interclass correlation reported

4. Timed Up and Go Test (TUG)

- **Description**: This functional mobility test measures the time taken for an individual to stand up from a chair, walk three meters, turn around, walk back, and sit down.
- **Purpose**: It assesses mobility and balance in a dynamic context.
- **Advantages**: Simple to administer and effective in predicting fall risk among older adults

5. Berg Balance Scale (BBS)

- **Description**: A widely used clinical tool that consists of 14 tasks assessing various aspects of balance through functional movements.
- **Scoring**: Each task is scored from 0 to 4, with higher scores indicating better balance.
- **Advantages**:
    - Good reliability and validity in assessing balance among older adults.
    - Comprehensive in evaluating multiple dimensions of balance

Conclusion

These self-assessment tools provide valuable insights into an individual's balance capabilities and potential fall risks. Regular use can help identify issues early, allowing for timely interventions aimed at improving stability and reducing the likelihood of falls.

Some Common scenarios that highlight personal balance challenges

Common scenarios that highlight personal balance challenges often stem from the interplay between work demands and personal life commitments. Here are some key areas where individuals frequently struggle to maintain balance:

Unrealistic Demands

Workplace Pressures: Many individuals face unreasonable expectations at work, such as excessive workloads, tight deadlines, and constant overtime. These pressures can lead to burnout and a feeling of being overwhelmed, making it difficult to manage personal responsibilities effectively

.Personal Commitments: On the personal front, family obligations can also impose unrealistic demands. For example, parents may find themselves juggling their children's activities while trying to meet work commitments, leading to conflicts and stress

Lack of Control

Inflexible Work Environments: A significant challenge arises when individuals feel they have little control over their schedules or workloads. This can manifest in unpredictable work hours or the inability to take time off when needed, contributing to stress and a sense of helplessness

.**Personal Life Events**: Situations such as illness or family emergencies can also create a sense of losing control, further complicating the balance between work and personal life

Unsupportive Relationships

Workplace Isolation: Unsupportive colleagues or management can exacerbate stress levels. When employees do not receive recognition or support, it can lead to feelings of isolation and dissatisfaction at work

.**Home Dynamics**: Similarly, unsupportive relationships at home—where family members may not understand or accommodate each other's needs—can create additional strain and hinder efforts to achieve balance

High Stress Levels

Overlapping Responsibilities: The accumulation of stress from both work and personal life can lead to high overall stress levels. This often results in physical symptoms like fatigue and emotional issues such as anxiety or depression, making it harder to maintain a healthy balance

Neglected Personal Time

Work Over Personal Life: When work demands encroach on personal time—such as skipping family events or neglecting hobbies—individuals may feel unfulfilled outside of their professional roles. This neglect can lead to decreased job satisfaction and overall well-being

Constant Multitasking

Juggling Multiple Roles: Many people find themselves constantly multitasking between work duties and personal responsibilities. This juggling act can reduce focus and efficiency, leading to increased stress and a diminished sense of accomplishment in both areas

Conclusion

Recognizing these common scenarios is crucial for individuals seeking to improve their work-life balance. Addressing these challenges often requires proactive strategies such as setting boundaries, improving communication, and prioritizing self-care. By understanding the sources of imbalance, individuals can take steps toward achieving a more harmonious integration of their professional and personal lives.

◈ Encouragement towards logging experiences and symptoms.

◈ Logging experiences and symptoms can be a powerful tool for individuals seeking to understand their health and well-being better. Here are several key points that highlight the importance and benefits of maintaining such records:

◈ Understanding Symptoms

◈ **Identification of Patterns**: Keeping a symptom diary allows individuals to track when symptoms occur, their duration, and any potential triggers. This can lead to a better understanding of personal health patterns, which is crucial for managing chronic conditions or identifying new health issues

◈ 1[1]

◈ .**Facilitating Diagnosis**: A detailed log can provide valuable information to healthcare providers, aiding in diagnosis and treatment planning. By documenting symptoms over time, patients can present a clearer picture of their health status during medical consultations

---

1. https://www.medicalnewstoday.com/articles/symptom-diary

Empowerment and Control

◊ **Increased Awareness**: Regularly logging experiences can empower individuals by increasing their awareness of their health. This proactive approach fosters a sense of control over one's well-being, allowing for more informed decisions regarding lifestyle changes or treatment options

◊ .**Management of Conditions**: For those with existing health conditions, tracking symptoms can help identify what alleviates or exacerbates their issues. This insight can lead to more effective self-management strategies, enhancing overall quality of life

Emotional and Mental Health Benefits

◊ **Reduction of Anxiety**: Documenting symptoms can alleviate anxiety related to uncertainty about one's health. Knowing that there is a systematic way to monitor changes can provide reassurance

◊ 1^2

◊ .**Reflection and Insight**: Logging experiences not only pertains to physical symptoms but can also include emotional states. This reflective practice can help individuals recognize stressors or emotional triggers, contributing to better mental health management

Practical Considerations

◊ **Variety of Formats**: Individuals can choose various methods for logging, from traditional notebooks to digital apps. This flexibility allows for personalized approaches that suit individual preferences and lifestyles

◊ .**Encouragement of Professional Consultation**: Keeping a symptom diary encourages individuals to seek professional help when necessary. If significant changes or concerning

---

2. https://www.medicalnewstoday.com/articles/symptom-diary

patterns emerge in the logs, it serves as a prompt to consult healthcare professionals promptly

⬦ .In conclusion, logging experiences and symptoms is an effective strategy for enhancing personal health management. It provides clarity, fosters empowerment, and supports better communication with healthcare providers, ultimately leading to improved well-being.

Importance of understanding triggers and patterns

⬦ Understanding the triggers and patterns of balance problems is crucial for several reasons, particularly in the context of health management and fall prevention.

1. Identification of Underlying Causes

⬦ **Medical Conditions**: Balance issues can stem from various medical conditions such as neurological disorders (e.g., Parkinson's disease, multiple sclerosis) or inner ear problems (e.g., vestibular disorders) that disrupt the vestibular system's function

⬦ Recognizing specific triggers can help healthcare providers diagnose underlying issues more effectively.

⬦ **Medication Effects**: Many medications can cause dizziness or balance impairments. Identifying which medications contribute to balance problems allows for better management and potential adjustments to treatment plans

2. Tailored Interventions

◇ **Personalized Treatment Plans**: Understanding individual patterns of balance issues enables healthcare providers to create targeted rehabilitation strategies. For instance, if a patient experiences balance problems during specific activities, tailored exercises can be designed to improve stability in those contexts

◇ **Behavioral Modifications**: Recognizing triggers such as environmental factors (e.g., uneven surfaces) or lifestyle choices (e.g., sedentary behavior) can lead to practical changes that enhance safety and reduce fall risk

3. Fall Prevention

◇ **Risk Assessment**: By identifying the specific triggers and patterns associated with balance problems, individuals and healthcare providers can assess fall risk more accurately. This is especially important for older adults, where falls are a leading cause of injury

◇ **Proactive Measures**: Understanding when and why balance issues occur allows for proactive measures, such as implementing home modifications or engaging in preventative exercises like Tai Chi, which have been shown to improve balance and reduce fall risk

4. Enhancing Quality of Life

◇ **Psychological Impact**: Awareness of triggers can help mitigate fear of falling, which often exacerbates balance issues. Addressing psychological factors associated with balance problems can lead to improved confidence and participation in daily activities

◈ **Social Engagement**: Balance impairments can limit social interactions and physical activities. By understanding and addressing these issues, individuals may feel more empowered to engage in community activities, thereby enhancing their overall quality of life

◈ In summary, understanding the triggers and patterns of balance problems is vital for effective diagnosis, tailored interventions, fall prevention strategies, and improving the overall quality of life for individuals affected by these issues.

Chapter 4: Seeking Help: When and Where

1

Guidance on when to consult a healthcare professional.

When experiencing balance problems, knowing when to consult a healthcare professional is crucial for effective diagnosis and treatment. Balance issues can stem from various underlying conditions, and timely medical intervention can significantly improve outcomes.

When to Seek Help

1. Persistent Symptoms:

- If you experience ongoing balance issues that last for more than a few days, it's advisable to consult a healthcare provider. This includes feelings of dizziness, unsteadiness, or frequent falls
- **2. Severe Dizziness:**

Seek immediate medical attention if dizziness is so severe that it impairs your ability to walk or drive safely

This could indicate a serious underlying condition.

3. Associated Symptoms:

- Consult a doctor if you experience additional symptoms such as:
  - Blurred vision
  - Confusion or disorientation
  - Lightheadedness or fainting spells
  - A sensation of spinning (vertigo) or feeling as if you are moving while stationary

4. Recent Injuries:

- If balance problems arise after a fall, car accident, or head injury, this constitutes a medical emergency and requires immediate evaluation

5. Medication Side Effects:

- If you suspect that your balance issues may be related to medications you're taking, discuss this with your healthcare provider. They may need to adjust your prescriptions**6. Age-Related Concerns:**

- Older adults should be particularly vigilant; if you are over 65 and notice changes in your balance or experience falls, seeking an evaluation is essential to prevent further complications
- Diagnostic Process

Healthcare providers typically begin with a thorough medical history and physical examination. They may perform various tests, including:

- **Balance Tests:** To assess stability and coordination.
- **Blood Tests:** To rule out infections or other systemic issues.
- **Imaging Tests:** Such as X-rays or MRIs to check for structural problems in the brain or inner earTreatment Options

Treatment for balance disorders varies based on the underlying cause but may include:

- **Vestibular Rehabilitation Therapy:** A specialized form of physical therapy aimed at improving balance through targeted exercises
- **Medication Management:** Adjusting medications that may contribute to dizziness or unsteadiness.

- **Lifestyle Modifications:** Recommendations may include dietary changes, hydration strategies, and exercises to strengthen muscles involved in balanceIn summary, if you are experiencing any concerning symptoms related to balance, particularly if they are persistent or severe, consulting a healthcare professional is essential for proper diagnosis and treatment.

2

Types of specialists who can help (e.g., audiologists, neurologists).

When dealing with vertigo, a variety of specialists can provide effective treatment based on the underlying cause. Here are the primary types of healthcare professionals who can help:

Types of Specialists

1. Neurologists:

- Neurologists are often the first point of contact for diagnosing and treating vertigo, especially when it is associated with neurological conditions. They can assess issues related to the brain and nervous system that may contribute to balance disorders. They may prescribe medications like antihistamines or perform tests to determine the cause of vertigo

2 Otolaryngologists (ENT Specialists):

- They manage conditions like Benign Paroxysmal Positional Vertigo (BPPV) through maneuvers such as the Epley maneuver. They also provide vestibular rehabilitation therapy to improve balance.Ear, Nose, and Throat (ENT) specialists diagnose and treat disorders related to the inner ear, which is crucial for balance. They can address conditions like Menière's disease, labyrinthitis, and other inner ear problems that may cause vertigo

4. Physical Therapists

- Physical therapists, particularly those trained in vestibular rehabilitation, develop exercise programs tailored to improve balance and reduce dizziness. They focus on strengthening muscles used for stability and coordination

5. Psychiatrists/Psychologists:

- In cases where vertigo has a psychological component or is exacerbated by anxiety, mental health professionals can provide therapy or medication to help manage these symptoms
- **6. Neuro-Otologists:**

- These specialists bridge the gap between neurology and otology, focusing specifically on disorders of the inner ear and their neurological implications. They are particularly adept at diagnosing complex cases of vertigoConclusion

Consulting the appropriate specialist based on your symptoms and medical history is essential for effective management of vertigo. Each type of specialist plays a unique role in diagnosing and treating the various causes of balance disorders, ensuring a comprehensive approach to care.

3

What to expect during a consultation and typical assessment protocols.

During a consultation for vertigo, patients can expect a comprehensive evaluation process that involves several steps to accurately diagnose the condition. Here's what typically happens during such an appointment:

Initial Consultation

1. Medical History:

- The healthcare provider will start by taking a detailed medical history. This includes questions about the nature of your symptoms, their onset, duration, and frequency, as well as any triggers you may have noticed. Be prepared to discuss:
  - Specific symptoms (e.g., spinning sensation, imbalance)
  - Recent injuries or illnesses
  - Medications you are currently taking

2. Symptom Assessment:

- You will be asked to describe your symptoms in detail. Common questions include:
  - When did the symptoms start?
  - Do they come and go or are they constant?
  - Are there specific movements or activities that trigger your symptoms?Physical Examination

3. Neurological Examination:

- The provider may conduct a neurological exam to assess coordination, reflexes, and balance. This helps determine if the vertigo is related to the nervous system
- **4. Balance Tests:**

- Various tests may be performed to evaluate your balance and vestibular function, including:
  - **Dix-Hallpike Maneuver:** To check for BPPV by observing eye movements as your head is moved into different positions.
  - **Electronystagmography (ENG) or Videonystagmography (VNG):** These tests measure

involuntary eye movements to assess inner ear function.This is done in relevant cases

- ○ **Vestibular Evoked Myogenic Potentials (VEMP):** To evaluate how well certain parts of your inner ear are functioningAdditional Testing

5. Imaging Tests:

- If necessary, imaging studies such as an MRI may be ordered to rule out other potential causes of vertigo, like tumors or structural abnormalities in the brain

Discussing Results and Next Steps

6. Diagnosis Discussion:

- After completing the assessments, the healthcare provider will discuss the findings with you. They will explain any diagnoses made and what they imply regarding your condition.

7. Treatment Options:

- Depending on the diagnosis, treatment options may include:
- **Epley's maneuver or Semont's maneuver** in BPPV which is the most common cause for vertigo

  - ○ **Vestibular Rehabilitation Therapy:** Exercises designed to improve balance.

  - ○ **Medications:** To alleviate symptoms or treat underlying conditions.

  - ○ **Lifestyle Modifications:** Such as dietary changes for conditions like Menière's disease

4

Resources for finding specialists and support groups

Finding specialists and support groups for vertigo can significantly enhance your understanding and management of the condition. Here are some valuable resources:

Resources for Finding Specialists

1. Vestibular Disorders Association (VEDA):

- VEDA provides a comprehensive directory of vestibular specialists, including audiologists, neurologists, and ENT specialists. Their website also offers educational resources about vestibular disorders, making it a great starting point for finding qualified professionals in your area. You can access their resources at vestibular.org
- **2. National Institute on Deafness and Other Communication Disorders (NIDCD):**

- The NIDCD offers information about vestibular disorders and can guide you to relevant specialists and treatment options. They provide a list of organizations that focus on balance disorders, which can help you connect with healthcare providers

Support Groups
1. Online Support Groups:

- Many online platforms host support groups specifically for individuals dealing with dizziness and vertigo. Facebook groups such as the **Vestibular Disorders Support Group, Vertigo Support Group,** and **Dizzy and Vertigo Support Group** allow members to share experiences, coping strategies, and emotional support
- **2. Local Chapters of VEDA:**

- VEDA also lists local chapters that may have in-person or virtual support groups. These groups provide a safe space for individuals to discuss their experiences and learn from others facing similar challenges

- **3. Community Centers and Hospitals:**

- Many community health centers or hospitals offer support groups for patients with vestibular disorders. Contact local healthcare facilities to inquire about available resources.

Additional Resources
1. Conferences and Workshops:

- Organizations like VEDA often host virtual conferences where patients can learn from experts about managing vestibular disorders. These events also provide opportunities to connect with other patients

2. Educational Materials:

- Many associations provide brochures, articles, and online resources that can help you understand your condition better and find appropriate care.

By utilizing these resources, individuals experiencing vertigo can find both professional help and community support, which are essential for effective management of their symptoms

Chapter 5: Treatment Options Explained

- Overview of various treatments available (e.g., medications, therapies).

Patients experiencing vertigo can benefit from a variety of treatments, including medications and therapies tailored to the underlying cause of their symptoms. Here's an overview of the available options:

Medications

1. Vestibular Suppressants:

- **Anticholinergics:** Medications like scopolamine are used to decrease vestibular system activity and alleviate symptoms

Antihistamines: Drugs such as meclizine and promethazine are effective for motion sickness and vertigo, helping to reduce nausea and dizziness

Benzodiazepines: These include diazepam and alprazolam, which can help manage anxiety-related vertigo but may have sedative effects

2. Specific Treatments for Conditions:

- **Ménière's Disease:** Treatment often involves a low-salt diet and diuretics to reduce fluid retention, along with vestibular suppressants during acute episodes

Vestibular Neuritis: Short-term use of vestibular suppressants is recommended, but physical therapy is crucial for recovery

Migraine-Associated Vertigo: Prophylactic medications like beta-blockers and calcium channel antagonists are commonly used

3. Anti-Nausea Medications:

- Drugs such as prochlorperazine and metoclopramide can help manage nausea associated with vertigo episodes

Therapies

1. Vestibular Rehabilitation Therapy (VRT):

- This physical therapy approach involves exercises designed to improve balance and reduce dizziness by retraining the brain to process vestibular information more effectively

2. Canalith Repositioning Maneuvers:

- Techniques like the Epley maneuver are specifically effective for benign paroxysmal positional vertigo (BPPV), helping to reposition displaced calcium crystals in the inner ear

3. Psychological Support:

- For patients whose vertigo is linked to anxiety disorders, psychotherapy may be beneficial in managing both anxiety and associated dizziness

Surgical Options

In rare cases where other treatments fail, surgical interventions may be considered, such as:

- **Gentamicin Injections: or steroid intratympanic administration**

To disable balance function in one ear, allowing the other ear to compensate.

- **Surgical Removal of Inner Ear Structures:** This is a last resort for severe cases of Ménière's disease or other debilitating conditions

Summary

The treatment of vertigo is multifaceted, involving a combination of medications tailored to specific conditions and various therapeutic approaches aimed at improving balance and reducing symptoms. A comprehensive assessment by healthcare professionals is essential for determining the most appropriate treatment plan based on individual patient needs.

Delving into physical therapy exercises tailored for balance improvement.

For individuals experiencing vertigo, physical therapy exercises can significantly improve balance and reduce symptoms. Here's an overview of effective exercises tailored for balance improvement in vertigo patients.

Key Physical Therapy Exercises

1. **Romberg Exercise**

- **Description:** Stand with your feet together and arms at your sides.
- **Goal:** Hold this position for at least 30 seconds. Progress by trying it with your eyes closed.
- **Frequency:** Perform twice daily until you can maintain balance without visual cues
- 2. **Standing Sway Exercise**

- **Forward and Backward Sway:**
    - Stand with feet shoulder-width apart.
    - Gently lean forward and backward, shifting weight from toes to heels without lifting your feet.
    - Aim for 20 repetitions.
- **Side-to-Side Sway:**
    - In the same stance, sway side to side.
    - Again, aim for 20 repetitions while ensuring your shoulders and hips move together
        - 3. Marching in Place

- **Description:** Stand with feet apart and arms at your sides.
- **Goal:** March in place, lifting knees high towards the ceiling.
- **Frequency:** Start with 20 steps, gradually increasing to 30. Try progressing to doing this exercise with your eyes closed
- 4. **Head Movements While Standing**

- While maintaining a comfortable standing position, perform the following head movements:
    - Up and down: 10 times
    - Side to side: 10 times
    - Diagonal movements: 10 times each direction
- This helps stimulate the vestibular system and improve spatial awareness
- 5. **Tandem Stance**

- **Description:** Stand with one foot directly in front of the other, as if on a tightrope.
- **Progression:** Start by holding onto a wall or chair for support. Gradually reduce support as balance improves. Switch foot positions regularly

6. Single-Leg Stance

- Once comfortable with tandem stance, try standing on one leg for as long as possible.
- Progress by closing your eyes or performing head movements while balancing

Safety Tips

- Always start slowly and consider having someone nearby for support during exercises.

- Use a chair or wall for stability, especially when trying new movements.
- Gradually increase the duration and complexity of exercises as balance improves.

Summary

Incorporating these physical therapy exercises into a daily routine can enhance balance and reduce the impact of vertigo symptoms over time. Regular practice is essential for achieving noticeable improvements in stability and confidence while moving. Always consult with a healthcare professional before starting any new exercise regimen to ensure safety and appropriateness based on individual conditions.

- Home exercises and routines that can be integrated into daily life.

For individuals experiencing vertigo, integrating specific home exercises into daily routines can significantly improve balance and reduce symptoms. Here's a comprehensive overview of effective exercises that can be performed at home.

Home Exercises for Vertigo

1. Brandt-Daroff Exercises

- **How to Perform:**
  - Start sitting upright.
  - Lie down on one side with your nose pointed up at a 45-degree angle. Hold for 30 seconds or until vertigo subsides.
  - Return to the seated position and wait for another 30 seconds.
  - Repeat on the other side.
- **Frequency:** Perform this sequence five times, twice a day

Gaze Stabilization Exercises

- **How to Perform:**
  - ○ Keep your head still and move your eyes side to side, up and down, and diagonally. Aim for 10 repetitions in each direction.
  - ○ Focus on a stationary object while moving your head side to side and up and down.
- **Goal:** Helps retrain the brain to manage dizziness when moving

3. Romberg Exercise

- **How to Perform:**
  - ○ Stand with your feet together and arms at your sides.
  - ○ Hold this position for 30 seconds. Progress by trying it with your eyes closed.
- **Frequency:** Twice daily until you can maintain balance without visual cues4. **Standing Sway Exercise**

- **How to Perform:**
  - ○ Stand with feet shoulder-width apart and arms at your sides.
  - ○ Gently lean forward and backward, then side to side, shifting weight without lifting your feet.
- **Frequency:** Start with 30 seconds in each direction, twice daily, gradually increasing duration

5. Marching in Place

- **How to Perform:**
  - ○ Stand comfortably and march in place, lifting knees

high.
- **Frequency:** Start with 20 steps, progressing to 30. Try doing this exercise with your eyes closed as you improve
- 6. **Epley Maneuver (Home Version)**

- **How to Perform:**
  - Sit upright and turn your head 45 degrees to the affected side.
  - Lie back quickly until your shoulders are on the pillow; hold for 30 seconds.
  - Turn your head to the opposite side without lifting it; hold for another 30 seconds.
- **Frequency:** Repeat this maneuver once a day until symptoms resolve7. **Foster Maneuver (Half Somersault)**

- **How to Perform:**
  - Start by kneeling on the floor and look straight ahead.
  - Tuck your chin down toward your chest while bringing your head towards the floor.
  - Quickly raise your head while keeping it turned toward one side; hold until dizziness passes.
- **Frequency:** Repeat as needed, waiting at least 15 minutes between attempts
- Safety Tips

- Always perform exercises in a safe environment where you can hold onto something stable if needed.
- Start slowly, especially if you are new to these exercises, and consider having someone nearby for support during initial attempts.
- Gradually increase the complexity and duration of exercises

as balance improves.

Summary

Incorporating these home exercises into daily routines can help individuals manage vertigo more effectively. Regular practice is crucial for improving balance and reducing symptoms over time. Always consult a healthcare professional before starting new exercises, especially if you have underlying health conditions or concerns about safety.

Importance of a multidisciplinary approach

A multidisciplinary approach is essential in the management of vertigo due to the complex and multifactorial nature of the condition. This approach involves collaboration among various healthcare professionals, each contributing their expertise to provide comprehensive care. Here's an overview of the importance of this strategy:

Comprehensive Assessment

- **Diverse Expertise:** Vertigo can stem from various causes, including vestibular disorders, neurological issues, and even psychological factors. A team comprising otolaryngologists, neurologists, audiologists, physiotherapists, and psychologists can perform thorough assessments to accurately diagnose the underlying cause of vertigo

Tailored Diagnosis: Each specialist can conduct specific tests relevant to their field, such as vestibular function tests, imaging studies, and balance assessments. This collaborative effort ensures that all potential causes are considered, leading to a more accurate diagnosis

Individualized Treatment Plans

- **Customized Interventions:** A multidisciplinary team can develop individualized treatment plans that address the unique needs of each patient. For example, while an otolaryngologist may focus on medical management or surgical options for inner ear disorders, a physiotherapist can design vestibular rehabilitation exercises tailored to improve balance and reduce symptoms

Holistic Care: This approach allows for the integration of various treatment modalities, including medication management, physical therapy, dietary changes, and psychological support. Such comprehensive care can enhance overall patient outcomes and quality of life

Enhanced Patient Education and Support

- **Patient-Centered Care:** Multidisciplinary teams can provide consistent education about vertigo and its management across different specialties. This ensures that patients receive clear information regarding their condition and treatment options from multiple perspectives

Support Systems: Collaboration among healthcare providers fosters a supportive environment for patients. Regular communication between team members allows for adjustments in treatment based on patient progress and feedback, ensuring that care remains responsive to individual needs

Improved Outcomes

- **Evidence-Based Practices:** Multidisciplinary approaches are often grounded in evidence-based practices that have been shown to yield better outcomes for patients with vertigo. Studies indicate that coordinated care can lead to reduced symptoms, improved balance, and enhanced daily functioning

Reduced Healthcare Costs: By addressing vertigo comprehensively from the outset, multidisciplinary care may prevent complications or the need for more extensive interventions later on. This proactive approach can ultimately reduce healthcare costs associated with recurrent visits or hospitalizations due to unmanaged symptoms

Conclusion

The complexity of vertigo necessitates a multidisciplinary approach to ensure effective management. By leveraging the expertise of various healthcare professionals, patients receive comprehensive assessments, individualized treatment plans, consistent education, and improved health outcomes. This collaborative model not only enhances patient care but also addresses the multifaceted nature of vertigo more effectively than any single discipline could achieve alone.

Chapter 6: Mind-Body Connection in Balance

- Exploring how stress and anxiety affect balance.

Stress and anxiety significantly impact balance, primarily through their effects on the vestibular system and overall motor control. Here's a detailed exploration of how these psychological factors influence balance:

Effects of Stress and Anxiety on Balance

1. **Physiological Responses**

   - **Hormonal Changes:** Stress triggers the release of hormones like cortisol, which can impair vestibular function. Elevated cortisol levels may disrupt neural transmission within the vestibular system, leading to difficulties in maintaining balance
   - **Muscle Tension:** Chronic stress often results in increased muscle tension, particularly in the neck and shoulders. This tension can affect posture and stability, making it harder for individuals to maintain balance

2. **Altered Motor Control**

   - **Increased Stiffness:** Anxiety can lead to stiffening of movements as individuals become hyper-aware of their surroundings. This rigidity may hinder fluid motion and response to balance challenges

Changes in Gait: Individuals with anxiety often modify their gait due to fear of falling. They may walk more slowly, widen their stance, or hesitate before stepping, which can further compromise balance and increase the risk of falls

3. Cognitive Effects

- **Impaired Concentration:** Anxiety can cloud cognitive functions, making it difficult for individuals to focus on tasks that require balance. This impairment can lead to misjudgments about spatial awareness and movement coordination

Fear of Falling: The fear associated with potential falls can create a vicious cycle where anxiety leads to reduced mobility, which in turn increases the risk of falling due to lack of practice and confidence in balance

4. Behavioral Changes

- **Avoidance Strategies:** People experiencing anxiety may avoid situations that require balance, such as walking on uneven surfaces or participating in physical activities. This avoidance can lead to deconditioning and further deterioration of balance skills over time

Visual Fixation: Anxious individuals might fixate on obstacles or hazards rather than maintaining a broader spatial awareness. This behavior can impair their ability to navigate environments safely, increasing the likelihood of accidents

Clinical Implications

Understanding the relationship between stress, anxiety, and balance is crucial for effective management:

- **Rehabilitation Programs:** Incorporating psychological assessments into rehabilitation can help address the underlying anxiety that contributes to balance issues. Tailoring physical therapy exercises to include stress-reduction techniques may enhance recovery outcomes
- **Holistic Treatment Approaches:** A multidisciplinary approach involving mental health professionals can provide

strategies for managing anxiety alongside physical rehabilitation, improving both psychological well-being and physical stability.

Conclusion

Stress and anxiety profoundly affect balance through physiological changes, altered motor control, cognitive impairments, and behavioral adaptations. Recognizing these connections is vital for developing comprehensive treatment plans that address both the psychological and physical aspects of vertigo and balance disorders. Effective management requires collaboration among healthcare providers to ensure holistic care that promotes recovery and enhances quality of life.

- Techniques for mindfulness and relaxation that promote stability.

Mindfulness and relaxation techniques can significantly enhance stability and balance, particularly for individuals experiencing vertigo or related balance disorders. By promoting a calm mind and body, these practices help mitigate the effects of stress and anxiety, which can negatively impact balance. Here's an exploration of effective techniques that can be integrated into daily life:

Techniques for Mindfulness and Relaxation

1. **Breathing Techniques**

- **Deep Breathing:** Focus on taking slow, deep breaths to stimulate the parasympathetic nervous system, promoting relaxation. Inhale deeply through the nose, allowing the abdomen to expand, then exhale slowly through the mouth.

- **Box Breathing:** This technique involves inhaling for four counts, holding for four counts, exhaling for four counts, and holding again for four counts. This structured breathing helps calm the mind and body.

2. Meditation Practices

- **Guided Meditation:** Listening to guided meditations can help individuals relax while providing structure to their mindfulness practice. Techniques like Yoga Nidra encourage deep relaxation while maintaining awareness.
- **Body Scan Meditation:** This involves systematically focusing attention on different parts of the body, noticing sensations, and releasing tension. It enhances body awareness and promotes relaxation.

3. Mindful Movement

- **Walking Meditation:** Practicing walking meditation encourages awareness of each step, the sensations in your feet, and your surroundings. This practice helps improve balance by fostering a connection between movement and mindfulness.
- **Gentle Yoga or Tai Chi:** These practices combine physical movement with mindfulness, enhancing flexibility and stability while promoting relaxation.

4. Nature Connection

- **Mindful Hiking:** Engaging with nature through mindful hiking allows individuals to focus on the sensory experiences of walking—like the texture of the ground or the sounds of nature—while reducing stress.

- **Nature Immersion:** Spending time outdoors can help ground individuals in the present moment, promoting a sense of calm and stability.

5. Visualization Techniques

- **Guided Imagery:** Visualizing a peaceful scene or imagining oneself successfully navigating challenging situations can reduce anxiety and enhance confidence in balance.
- **Mountain Meditation:** This technique involves visualizing oneself as a mountain—stable and unmovable—promoting a sense of strength and grounding.

6. Mindful Eating and Drinking

- Paying attention to the sensory experiences involved in eating or drinking—such as taste, texture, and temperature—can enhance mindfulness in everyday activities. This practice encourages presence in the moment and reduces stress.

7. Stretching and Relaxation Exercises

- Gentle stretching can be performed mindfully to release tension in muscles that affect balance. Focus on breathing deeply during stretches to enhance relaxation.
- Progressive muscle relaxation involves tensing and then relaxing different muscle groups while focusing on breath, helping to alleviate physical tension.

8. Mindful Observation

- Practicing mindful observation involves focusing on objects in your environment without judgment. This could include gazing at a candle flame or observing nature, which helps cultivate concentration and calmness.

Conclusion

Incorporating mindfulness and relaxation techniques into daily routines can significantly promote stability by reducing stress and anxiety levels that adversely affect balance. These practices foster greater body awareness, enhance mental clarity, and improve overall well-being. Regular engagement with these techniques not only aids in managing vertigo but also contributes to a more balanced life overall.

1. Improved Proprioception

- **Body Awareness:** Yoga emphasizes body awareness through various poses that require individuals to focus on their alignment and posture. This heightened awareness enhances proprioception, which is crucial for maintaining balance.

2. Strengthening Core Muscles

- **Core Stability:** Many yoga poses engage core muscles, which play a vital role in stabilizing the body. A strong core helps maintain balance during dynamic movements and reduces the risk of falls.

3. Flexibility and Range of Motion

- **Increased Flexibility:** Yoga promotes flexibility through stretching, which can improve joint mobility. Greater flexibility allows for more fluid movements, contributing to better balance.

4. Focus on Breath Control

- **Calming Effects:** Breath control techniques in yoga help reduce anxiety and stress, which can otherwise impair balance. A calm mind allows for better concentration on maintaining stability during movements.

5. Mindfulness Practice

- **Mental Focus:** Yoga encourages mindfulness, helping practitioners stay present in the moment. This mental clarity is essential for executing movements with precision and maintaining balance.

Benefits of Tai Chi in Enhancing Balance and Coordination
1. Slow, Controlled Movements

- **Balance Training:** Tai Chi involves slow, deliberate movements that challenge balance and coordination without the risk of injury associated with high-impact exercises. This method allows practitioners to develop stability gradually.

2. Weight Shifting Techniques

- **Dynamic Balance:** The practice emphasizes shifting weight from one leg to another, which enhances dynamic balance and improves the ability to adapt to changing conditions while moving.

3. Integration of Mind and Body

- **Holistic Approach:** Tai Chi combines physical movement with mindfulness and breath control, fostering a holistic approach that enhances both physical stability and mental clarity.

4. Strengthening Lower Body Muscles

- **Leg Strength:** Many Tai Chi movements focus on strengthening the legs, which are critical for maintaining balance. Stronger leg muscles contribute to better stability during standing and walking.

5. Research Support

- Studies have shown that Tai Chi can significantly reduce the risk of falls among older adults by improving balance and coordination. For instance, a systematic review indicated that Tai Chi effectively decreases fall risk and enhances balance ability across various populations

Conclusion

Both yoga and Tai Chi offer valuable benefits for enhancing balance and coordination through their unique approaches to movement, strength building, flexibility, and mindfulness. Regular practice of these disciplines can lead to improved stability, reduced fall risk, and enhanced overall well-being. Integrating these practices into daily routines can be particularly beneficial for older adults or individuals recovering from injuries or experiencing balance issues.

- Practical tips for incorporating mindful practices into daily routines.
- Incorporating mindful practices into daily routines can significantly aid in the management of vertigo by reducing stress and enhancing overall well-being. Here are practical tips for integrating mindfulness and relaxation techniques into everyday life:
- Practical Tips for Mindful Practices
- 1. **Start with Breathing Exercises**
- **Deep Breathing:** Dedicate a few minutes each day to practice deep breathing. Inhale deeply through your nose, allowing your abdomen to expand, then exhale slowly through your mouth. This can help calm the nervous system.
- **Box Breathing:** Try inhaling for four counts, holding for four counts, exhaling for four counts, and holding again for four counts. Repeat this cycle several times.
- 2. **Engage in Yoga or Tai Chi**
- **Daily Yoga Routine:** Incorporate specific yoga poses beneficial for vertigo, such as Shanmukhi Mudra or Paschimottanasana. These poses promote relaxation and

improve balance.

- **Tai Chi Practice:** Spend 15-30 minutes practicing Tai Chi movements that emphasize slow, controlled motions to enhance stability and coordination.
- 3. **Mindful Walking**
- **Meditative Walking:** Take a daily walk while focusing on each step you take. Pay attention to the sensations in your feet and legs as you move. This practice helps ground you and improves balance.
- **Nature Walks:** If possible, walk in nature and engage your senses by noticing the sights, sounds, and smells around you.
- 4. **Incorporate Mindfulness into Daily Activities**
- **Mindful Eating:** Practice eating slowly and savoring each bite. Focus on the flavors, textures, and aromas of your food to enhance mindfulness during meals.
- **Mindful Drinking:** When enjoying a beverage, take time to appreciate its warmth or coolness, and notice how it feels as you sip.
- 5. **Practice Meditation Regularly**
- **Guided Meditation:** Use apps or online resources for guided meditation sessions that focus on relaxation and grounding.
- **Body Scan Meditation:** Spend a few minutes lying down or sitting comfortably while mentally scanning your body from head to toe, noticing any areas of tension and consciously relaxing them.
- 6. **Utilize Visualization Techniques**
- **Imagery for Calmness:** Visualize a peaceful scene or imagine yourself successfully navigating challenging situations. This can help reduce anxiety related to vertigo.

- **Mountain Meditation:** Picture yourself as a stable mountain, unmovable despite external pressures, fostering a sense of strength and grounding.
- 7. **Establish a Routine**
- **Set Aside Time Daily:** Designate specific times each day for mindfulness practices—whether it's morning meditation or evening yoga—to create consistency.
- **Combine Practices:** Consider integrating breathing exercises with yoga or Tai Chi sessions for a comprehensive approach.
- 8. **Use Technology Mindfully**
- **Mindfulness Apps:** Explore apps designed for mindfulness and meditation that offer guided sessions tailored to stress reduction and relaxation.
- **Limit Screen Time:** Be mindful of your screen time, especially before bed. Reducing exposure to screens can improve sleep quality and reduce anxiety.
- Conclusion
- Incorporating these mindful practices into daily routines can significantly contribute to managing vertigo symptoms by promoting relaxation, reducing stress, and enhancing balance. Regular engagement with these techniques fosters greater awareness of the body and mind, leading to improved well-being over time. Always consult with healthcare professionals before starting new practices to ensure they align with individual health needs.

Chapter 7: Nutrition and Balance

- Impact of diet on overall health and stability.

Diet plays a significant role in managing overall health and can be particularly impactful for individuals experiencing vertigo. Vertigo, characterized by a sensation of spinning or dizziness, often stems from issues within the vestibular system. Dietary adjustments can help mitigate symptoms and improve quality of life.

Key Dietary Strategies for Managing Vertigo

1. Nutrient-Dense Foods:

- **Fruits and Vegetables:** Rich in vitamins, minerals, antioxidants, and fiber, these foods are essential for maintaining overall health and supporting vestibular function. Leafy greens, broccoli, and peppers are particularly beneficial
- **Healthy Fats:** Foods high in omega-3 fatty acids, such as salmon and sardines, may help reduce inflammation and improve brain function

2. Hydration:

- **Water Intake:** Staying adequately hydrated is crucial as dehydration can lead to decreased blood volume and exacerbate dizziness. Aim for at least two liters of water daily

3. Balanced Meal Timing:

- **Regular Meal Schedule:** Establishing a consistent eating pattern helps stabilize blood glucose levels, reducing the likelihood of dizziness associated with fluctuations

Foods to Avoid
1. High Sugar Foods:

- Foods with high sugar content can lead to spikes and crashes in blood sugar levels, which may trigger vertigo symptoms

2. High Sodium Foods:

- Excessive sodium intake can worsen conditions like Meniere's disease, which is linked to severe vertigo episodes

3. Caffeine and Alcohol:

- These substances can affect hydration and contribute to balance issues, making them advisable to limit or avoid altogether

Supplementation

Incorporating supplements may also be beneficial for some individuals. Nutrients such as magnesium and vitamin B12 have been linked to improved vestibular health. However, it is essential to consult with a healthcare professional before starting any supplement regimen to avoid potential interactions with medications

Conclusion

A well-structured diet focusing on nutrient-dense foods while avoiding triggers can significantly impact the management of vertigo symptoms. Regular hydration, balanced meal timing, and careful selection of foods can enhance overall health stability and reduce the frequency of vertigo episodes. For personalized dietary advice tailored to individual health needs, consulting with a healthcare professional is recommended.

- Key nutrients and foods that support vestibular function.

Supporting vestibular function through diet involves incorporating specific nutrients and foods that enhance overall health and mitigate symptoms associated with vestibular disorders. Here are the key nutrients and foods beneficial for vestibular health:

Key Nutrients for Vestibular Function

1. Omega-3 Fatty Acids:

- Essential for reducing inflammation and supporting cell membrane integrity.
- Found in fatty fish like salmon, mackerel, sardines, and plant sources such as walnuts and flaxseeds.

2. Vitamins:

- **Vitamin B6:** Important for nerve function and can help alleviate symptoms of dizziness. Sources include chicken, fish, potatoes, and bananas.
- **Vitamin C:** Supports immune function and may improve blood circulation, which is vital for vestibular health. Rich sources include citrus fruits (oranges, lemons), strawberries, and bell peppers.
- **Vitamin D:** Crucial for bone health and may aid in maintaining inner ear balance. Foods high in vitamin D include fatty fish, egg yolks, fortified dairy products, and mushrooms.

- **Vitamin B12:** Necessary for neurological function; deficiencies can lead to balance issues. Found in animal products like meat, eggs, and dairy.

3. Minerals:

- **Magnesium:** Helps regulate nerve function and blood pressure, which are important for balance. Good sources include leafy greens (spinach, kale), nuts, seeds, and whole grains.
- **Zinc:** An antioxidant that supports immune function and may help reduce the risk of recurrent vertigo. Found in meats, shellfish, legumes, seeds, and nuts.

Foods to Include

Food Group	Examples	Key Nutrients
Fatty Fish	Salmon, mackerel, sardines	Omega-3 fatty acids, Vitamin D
Fruits	Oranges, strawberries, kiwis	Vitamin C
Vegetables	Spinach, broccoli, kale	Magnesium, Vitamins B6 & C
Legumes	Lentils, chickpeas	Protein, Magnesium
Nuts & Seeds	Walnuts, flaxseeds	Omega-3 fatty acids
Whole Grains	Quinoa, brown rice	B Vitamins
Dairy Products	Milk, yogurt	Calcium, Vitamin D

Additional Considerations

- **Hydration:** Maintaining proper hydration is crucial as

dehydration can exacerbate dizziness. Aim to drink plenty of water throughout the day.

- **Balanced Diet:** A varied diet rich in antioxidants from fruits and vegetables can help protect cells from damage.

Incorporating these nutrients and foods into daily meals can significantly support vestibular function and help manage symptoms associated with vestibular disorders. For personalized dietary advice or if you have specific health conditions related to vertigo or dizziness, consulting with a healthcare professional is advisable.

- Hydration and its role in maintaining physical stability.

Hydration is essential for maintaining physical stability and balance, playing a critical role in various bodily functions that directly impact overall health. Here's how adequate hydration contributes to maintaining balance:

Role of Hydration in Maintaining Physical Stability

1. Regulation of Body Temperature:

- Water helps regulate body temperature, especially during physical activity or in hot environments. Proper hydration allows for effective sweating, which cools the body and prevents overheating. This is crucial for maintaining physical performance and stability during exertion

2. Joint Lubrication:

- The cartilage in joints is composed of approximately 80% water. Adequate hydration ensures that joints remain well-lubricated, reducing friction and allowing for smoother movement. This lubrication helps prevent injuries and supports overall physical stability

3. Nutrient Transport:

- Water is vital for transporting nutrients, oxygen, and electrolytes throughout the body. Proper hydration ensures that muscles receive the necessary nutrients to function effectively, which is essential for maintaining strength and coordination
- **4. Muscle Function:**

- Dehydration can lead to muscle cramps, fatigue, and decreased strength, all of which can impair balance and coordination. Staying hydrated supports optimal muscle function, enhancing physical performance and stability during activities

5. Cognitive Function:

- Hydration significantly impacts brain function; even mild dehydration can impair memory, mood, and cognitive performance. Good hydration helps maintain focus and reaction times, which are critical for balance and stability
- **6. Cardiovascular Health:**

- Proper hydration helps maintain blood volume and pressure, ensuring efficient circulation. This is crucial for delivering oxygen to muscles and the brain, both of which are necessary for maintaining physical stability during movement

Recommendations for Hydration

- **Daily Intake:** It is commonly recommended to drink at least eight 8-ounce glasses of water daily, although individual needs may vary based on factors like activity level, climate, and health status
- **Hydration During Activity:** Drink water before, during, and after exercise to replenish fluids lost through sweat. This practice is especially important in hot or humid conditions where fluid loss can be significant
- **Listen to Your Body:** Pay attention to thirst cues and monitor urine color as indicators of hydration status.

In summary, maintaining adequate hydration is vital not only for overall health but also specifically for ensuring physical stability and balance. Proper fluid intake supports joint health, muscle function, cognitive performance, and cardiovascular efficiency—all essential components for maintaining stability during daily activities and exercise.

Sample meal plans and recipes for a balanced diet

Creating a balanced diet for individuals experiencing vertigo involves incorporating nutrient-dense foods while avoiding triggers that may exacerbate symptoms. Below is a sample meal plan along with recipes that focus on supporting vestibular function.

Sample Meal Plan for Vertigo Patients

Day 1

Breakfast:

- **Spinach and Mushroom Omelet**
  - Ingredients: 2 eggs, a handful of spinach, 1/2 cup mushrooms, salt, and pepper to taste.
  - Instructions: Sauté mushrooms and spinach in a non-stick skillet. Whisk eggs, pour them over the

vegetables, cook until set, then fold.

- **Whole Grain Avocado Toast**
  - ○ Ingredients: 1 slice whole grain bread, 1/2 avocado, lemon juice, salt, and pepper.
  - ○ Instructions: Mash avocado with lemon juice, salt, and pepper; spread on toasted bread.

Lunch:

- **Ground Turkey Chili**
  - ○ Ingredients: 1 lb ground turkey, 1 can kidney beans, 1 can diced tomatoes, chili powder, cumin.
  - ○ Instructions: Brown turkey in a pot, add beans and tomatoes, season with spices, simmer for 30 minutes.
- **Side Salad**
  - ○ Ingredients: Mixed greens, cherry tomatoes, cucumber, olive oil, and lemon dressing.

Dinner:

- **Grilled Salmon with Quinoa and Steamed Broccoli**
  - ○ Ingredients: 1 salmon fillet, 1 cup quinoa, broccoli florets.
  - ○ Instructions: Grill salmon until cooked through. Cook quinoa according to package instructions. Steam broccoli until tender.

Snacks:

- Greek yogurt with mixed berries and a sprinkle of chia seeds.
- A banana with almond butter.
- A handful of walnuts or dark chocolate.

Day 2

Breakfast:

- Berry Smoothie
    - Ingredients: 1 cup Greek yogurt, 1/2 cup mixed berries (strawberries, blueberries), a handful of spinach, and coconut water.
    - Instructions: Blend all ingredients until smooth.

Lunch:

- Chicken Salad
    - Ingredients: Grilled chicken breast, mixed greens (spinach and arugula), cherry tomatoes, sliced cucumber, almonds, olive oil dressing.

Dinner:

- Baked Cod with Sweet Potatoes and Asparagus
    - Ingredients: Cod fillet seasoned with herbs (dill or parsley), sweet potatoes (cubed), asparagus spears.
    - Instructions: Bake cod at 375°F for about 15 minutes. Roast sweet potatoes and asparagus on a baking sheet until tender.

Snacks:

- Carrot sticks with hummus.
- A small bowl of mixed nuts (almonds and hazelnuts).
- Sliced apple with peanut butter.

Key Nutritional Focus
Foods to Include

- **Leafy Greens:** Spinach and kale are rich in magnesium and B vitamins.

- **Fruits:** Berries and bananas provide antioxidants and potassium.
- **Healthy Fats:** Nuts and avocados support brain health.
- **Lean Proteins:** Chicken, turkey, fish (especially fatty fish like salmon) provide essential nutrients without excessive fat.

Foods to Avoid

- High-sodium foods that can lead to fluid retention.
- Caffeine and alcohol which can worsen symptoms of dizziness.
- Sugary snacks that may cause blood sugar fluctuations.

Conclusion

This meal plan emphasizes a balanced intake of nutrients beneficial for managing vertigo while avoiding potential triggers. Adjustments can be made based on individual preferences or dietary restrictions. Always consult with a healthcare professional or nutritionist for personalized dietary advice tailored to specific health needs.

Chapter 8: Creating a Safe Environment

- Home modifications to prevent falls and enhance safety.

To enhance safety for individuals with vertigo and prevent falls at home, several modifications can be implemented. These adjustments focus on creating a safer environment that accommodates the unique challenges faced by those experiencing balance issues.

Home Modifications for Fall Prevention

1. Improve Lighting:

- **Install Nightlights:** Place nightlights in hallways, bathrooms, and bedrooms to illuminate paths during nighttime
- **Use Motion-Sensor Lights:** These can help ensure that areas are well-lit when someone approaches, reducing the risk of tripping in dark spaces
- **2. Remove Hazards:**

- **Clear Clutter:** Keep floors free of obstacles such as shoes, books, and electrical cords to minimize tripping risks
- **Secure Rugs:** Use non-slip backing or remove loose rugs entirely to prevent slipping

3. Install Supportive Features:

- **Grab Bars:** Install grab bars in bathrooms near toilets and showers, as well as along stairways to provide additional support when standing or moving.
- **Handrails:** Ensure that all staircases have sturdy handrails on both sides

4. Optimize Furniture Arrangement:

- **Reorganize for Accessibility:** Arrange furniture to create clear pathways that allow for easy navigation without obstacles. Ensure that furniture is stable and at appropriate heights for sitting and standing

5. Flooring Considerations:

- **Choose Slip-Resistant Surfaces:** Install flooring that is slip-resistant and avoid materials like polished wood or tiles that can become slippery when wet
- **Remove Uneven Surfaces:** Repair any uneven flooring or steps that could pose a tripping hazard

6. Enhance Bathroom Safety:

- **Non-Slip Mats:** Use non-slip mats in the bathtub and shower to prevent falls during bathing
- **Raised Toilet Seats:** Consider installing raised toilet seats to make sitting down and getting up easier

7. Assistive Devices:

- **Walking Aids:** Encourage the use of walkers or canes if needed for additional stability while moving around the home

Personal Alarms: Consider using personal alarms that can alert others in case of a fall, providing peace of mind

8. Regular Health Assessments:

- **Consult Healthcare Providers:** Regular check-ups can help identify any underlying health issues contributing to dizziness or balance problems. Discuss any medications that may affect balance with a healthcare provider

Additional Strategies

- **Physical Activity:** Engage in exercises aimed at improving strength, balance, and flexibility, such as tai chi or supervised physical therapy programs. These activities can significantly reduce the risk of falls by enhancing overall stability
- **Vision Care:** Regular eye exams are crucial since poor vision can increase fall risks; ensure any vision issues are addressed promptly

By implementing these modifications and strategies, individuals with vertigo can create a safer living environment that minimizes the risk of falls and enhances their overall safety at home.

- Importance of clutter-free spaces and proper lighting.

Reducing visual clutter in the home is essential for creating a calm and organized environment. Here are some practical ways to achieve this:

Practical Ways to Reduce Visual Clutter

1. Designate a Place for Everything:

- Ensure that every item has a specific location. This habit encourages returning items to their designated spots, minimizing clutter buildup on surfaces.

2. Clear Surfaces:

- Keep tables, countertops, and other flat surfaces clear. This is one of the easiest ways to instantly reduce visual clutter and create a more spacious feel in any room

3. Use Organizers:

- Implement trays or bins to group small items together. This not only organizes but also visually contains clutter, making spaces look tidier

4. Limit Displayed Items:

- Choose only your favorite or most aesthetically pleasing items to display. Group them in odd numbers (like three or five) for a more visually appealing arrangement, while storing the rest out of sight

5. Create Uniformity:

- Use similar styles and colors for storage bins and labels. A cohesive color palette can make spaces feel more organized and less chaotic

6. Manage Cables:

- Conceal cables using cable management solutions like trunks or raceways. This prevents unsightly tangles from becoming a visual distraction

7. Utilize Vertical Space:

- Install shelves or use stackable storage solutions to keep items off the floor and surfaces. This not only saves space but also reduces visual clutter by drawing the eye upward

8. Declutter Regularly:

- Make it a habit to regularly assess your belongings, removing items that are no longer needed or loved. This ongoing practice helps maintain a clutter-free environment

9. Embrace Negative Space:

- Allow for empty spaces around displayed items to give the eyes a chance to rest. This approach can significantly reduce feelings of chaos in a room

10. Organize by Frequency of Use:

- Store frequently used items within easy reach while placing less-used items in less accessible areas. This strategic organization helps keep surfaces clear and functional

By implementing these strategies, individuals can effectively reduce visual clutter in their homes, leading to a more serene and organized living space that promotes well-being and ease of movement.

- Use of assistive devices and resources available.

Assistive devices and resources can significantly aid individuals experiencing vertigo, enhancing their safety and quality of life. Here are some key options available:

Assistive Devices

1. Mobility Aids:

- **Canes and Walkers:** These provide stability and support while walking, helping to prevent falls. They are particularly useful for those who feel unsteady or dizzy.
- **Grab Bars:** Installing grab bars in bathrooms and near stairs offers additional support when standing or moving, reducing the risk of slips.

2. Vestibular Rehabilitation Tools:

- **Balance Boards:** These can be used as part of vestibular rehabilitation therapy to improve balance and coordination.
- **Therapy Balls:** These help strengthen core muscles and improve stability, which can be beneficial for managing vertigo symptoms.

3. Home Modifications:

- **Non-Slip Mats:** Placing these in high-risk areas like bathrooms can prevent slips.
- **Lighting Solutions:** Motion-sensor lights or nightlights can help illuminate paths, reducing the risk of falls during nighttime.

Resources for Support and Treatment
1. Vestibular Rehabilitation Therapy (VRT):

- This specialized physical therapy focuses on exercises designed to improve balance and reduce dizziness. VRT may include maneuvers like the Epley maneuver, which helps reposition calcium crystals in the inner ear that cause benign paroxysmal positional vertigo (BPPV) **2. Professional Support:**

- **Physical Therapists:** Finding a therapist experienced in vestibular disorders can provide tailored treatment plans that include specific exercises to manage symptoms
- **Vestibular Disorders Association:** This organization offers resources to locate qualified therapists and information about managing vertigo
- **3. Medication:**

- Depending on the cause of vertigo, medications such as antihistamines, diuretics, or vestibular suppressants may be prescribed to alleviate symptoms

4. Educational Resources:

- Online platforms and local health services often provide educational materials about vertigo management, including lifestyle changes that can help reduce symptoms, such as dietary adjustments and stress management techniques Incorporating these assistive devices and utilizing available resources can empower individuals with vertigo to navigate their daily lives more safely and effectively, ultimately improving their overall well-bein Assessing and improving living conditions for individuals with vertigo is crucial for enhancing safety and reducing the risk of falls. Here's a comprehensive checklist to guide this process:

Checklist for Assessing and Improving Living Conditions for Vertigo Patients

1. Environmental Safety

- **Clear Walkways:**
    - Ensure all pathways are free of clutter, furniture, and obstacles.
    - Remove loose rugs or secure them with non-slip backing.
- **Install Grab Bars:**
    - Place grab bars in bathrooms (near toilets and showers) and along stairways.
- **Improve Lighting:**
    - Use bright, even lighting in all rooms, especially hallways and staircases.
    - Install motion-sensor lights or nightlights in key areas.

2. Furniture Arrangement

- **Stable Furniture:**
    - Ensure all furniture is sturdy and stable.
    - Arrange furniture to create clear, wide paths for easy

navigation.

- **Limit Low Furniture:**
    - ○ Avoid low tables or furniture that may pose a tripping hazard.

3. Bathroom Modifications

- **Non-Slip Mats:**
    - ○ Use non-slip mats in the bathtub and shower.
- **Raised Toilet Seats:**
    - ○ Consider installing raised toilet seats to make sitting down and standing up easier.

4. Bedroom Safety

- **Bed Height:**
    - ○ Ensure the bed is at a height that allows easy access without straining.
- **Nightstand Accessibility:**
    - ○ Keep essential items within reach from the bed (e.g., water, phone).

5. Kitchen Safety

- **Organized Storage:**
    - ○ Store frequently used items at waist level to avoid reaching or bending.
- **Avoid Climbing:**
    - ○ Use a sturdy step stool with handrails if needed; avoid using unstable chairs to reach high items.

6. Mobility Aids

- **Assess Need for Aids:**
  - Evaluate whether walking aids (canes, walkers) are necessary for stability.
- **Use of Shoes:**
  - Encourage wearing well-fitting, non-slip shoes indoors and outdoors.

7. Emergency Preparedness

- **Personal Alarm Systems:**
  - Consider a personal emergency response system (PERS) that can alert others in case of a fall.
- **Emergency Contacts:**
  - Keep a list of emergency contacts easily accessible.

8. Health Management

- **Regular Check-ups:**
  - Schedule regular appointments with healthcare providers to manage vertigo symptoms effectively.
- **Medication Review:**
  - Review medications with a healthcare professional to identify any that may exacerbate vertigo symptoms.

9. Lifestyle Adjustments

- **Hydration and Nutrition:**
  - Encourage adequate hydration and a balanced diet rich in vitamins and minerals.
- **Stress Management Techniques:**
  - Incorporate relaxation techniques such as deep

breathing or meditation to reduce stress, which can worsen vertigo symptoms.

10. Education and Support

- **Inform Family Members:**
  - Educate family members about vertigo management strategies and how they can assist.
- **Support Groups:**
  - Consider joining support groups for individuals with vertigo to share experiences and coping strategies.

Implementing this checklist can significantly enhance the living conditions for individuals with vertigo, promoting safety, comfort, and overall quality of life.

Answer

Creating a vertigo-friendly home environment involves several key components that prioritize safety, accessibility, and comfort. Here are the essential elements to consider:

Key Components of a Vertigo-Friendly Home Environment

1. Safe Flooring

- **Slip-Resistant Surfaces:** Use flooring materials that provide good traction, such as non-slip vinyl or rubber flooring. Avoid carpets with thick padding or loose rugs that can cause tripping hazards
- **Level Surfaces:** Ensure all walking surfaces are firm and even, minimizing the risk of unexpected changes in elevation

2. Adequate Lighting

- **Bright and Even Lighting:** Install bright, non-flickering lights throughout the home to improve visibility. This includes using energy-efficient bulbs and ensuring that light switches are easily accessible
- **Nightlights and Motion Sensors:** Place nightlights in hallways and bathrooms, and consider motion-sensor lights to illuminate paths during nighttime

3. Clutter-Free Spaces

- **Clear Walkways:** Keep all pathways free from clutter, furniture, and obstacles to allow for safe navigation. Regularly assess areas for potential tripping hazards like loose items or uneven surfaces

- **Organized Storage:** Use storage solutions like bins and trays to keep items organized and out of sight, reducing visual clutter that can overwhelm individuals with vestibular disorders

4. Supportive Furniture

- **Sturdy Seating:** Choose chairs and beds that are easy to get in and out of, with armrests for added support. Avoid low furniture that may require bending down too far
- **Grab Bars:** Install grab bars in key areas such as bathrooms, near toilets, and in hallways to provide additional support when standing or moving

5. Bathroom Safety

- **Non-Slip Mats:** Use non-slip mats in the shower and around the toilet to prevent slips
- **Raised Toilet Seats:** Consider installing raised toilet seats to assist with sitting down and standing up more easily

6. Emergency Preparedness

- **Personal Alarm Systems:** Implement a personal emergency response system (PERS) that allows individuals to alert others in case of a fall or emergency
- **Accessible Exits:** Ensure multiple exits from the home are clear and easy to navigate in case of emergencies

7. Health Management Resources

- **Regular Health Check-ups:** Schedule routine appointments with healthcare providers to monitor vertigo symptoms and adjust treatment as necessary
- **Vestibular Rehabilitation Therapy (VRT):** Consider engaging in VRT to improve balance and reduce dizziness through targeted exercises

8. Environmental Adjustments

- **Minimize Noise and Glare:** Use soundproofing techniques if necessary, and reduce glare from windows with sheer blinds or curtains to create a more comfortable environment
- **Simplified Décor:** Opt for simple patterns and neutral colors in furnishings to avoid overwhelming visual stimuli that can trigger symptoms

By incorporating these components into the home environment, individuals with vertigo can significantly enhance their safety, comfort, and overall quality of life.

Checklist for assessing and improving living conditions

Assessing and improving living conditions for individuals with vertigo is crucial for enhancing safety and reducing the risk of falls. Here's a comprehensive checklist to guide this process:

Checklist for Assessing and Improving Living Conditions for Vertigo Patients

1. Environmental Safety

- Clear Walkways:
    - Ensure all pathways are free of clutter, furniture, and obstacles.
    - Remove loose rugs or secure them with non-slip backing.
- Install Grab Bars:
    - Place grab bars in bathrooms (near toilets and showers) and along stairways.
- Improve Lighting:
    - Use bright, even lighting in all rooms, especially hallways and staircases.
    - Install motion-sensor lights or nightlights in key areas.

2. Furniture Arrangement

- Stable Furniture:
    - Ensure all furniture is sturdy and stable.
    - Arrange furniture to create clear, wide paths for easy navigation.
- Limit Low Furniture:
    - Avoid low tables or furniture that may pose a tripping hazard.

3. Bathroom Modifications

- **Non-Slip Mats:**
    - Use non-slip mats in the bathtub and shower.
- **Raised Toilet Seats:**
    - Consider installing raised toilet seats to make sitting down and standing up easier.

4. Bedroom Safety

- **Bed Height:**
    - Ensure the bed is at a height that allows easy access without straining.
- **Nightstand Accessibility:**
    - Keep essential items within reach from the bed (e.g., water, phone).

5. Kitchen Safety

- **Organized Storage:**
    - Store frequently used items at waist level to avoid reaching or bending.
- **Avoid Climbing:**
    - Use a sturdy step stool with handrails if needed; avoid using unstable chairs to reach high items.

6. Mobility Aids

- **Assess Need for Aids:**
    - Evaluate whether walking aids (canes, walkers) are necessary for stability.
- **Use of Shoes:**
    - Encourage wearing well-fitting, non-slip shoes indoors and outdoors.

7. Emergency Preparedness

- **Personal Alarm Systems:**
  - Consider a personal emergency response system (PERS) that can alert others in case of a fall.
- **Emergency Contacts:**
  - Keep a list of emergency contacts easily accessible.

8. Health Management

- **Regular Check-ups:**
  - Schedule regular appointments with healthcare providers to manage vertigo symptoms effectively.
- **Medication Review:**
  - Review medications with a healthcare professional to identify any that may exacerbate vertigo symptoms.

9. Lifestyle Adjustments

- **Hydration and Nutrition:**
  - Encourage adequate hydration and a balanced diet rich in vitamins and minerals.
- **Stress Management Techniques:**
  - Incorporate relaxation techniques such as deep breathing or meditation to reduce stress, which can worsen vertigo symptoms.

10. Education and Support

- **Inform Family Members:**
  - Educate family members about vertigo

management strategies and how they can assist.
- Support Groups:
  - Consider joining support groups for individuals with vertigo to share experiences and coping strategies.

Implementing this checklist can significantly enhance the living conditions for individuals with vertigo, promoting safety, comfort, and overall quality of life.
. Here are the essential elements to consider:
Key Components of a Vertigo-Friendly Home Environment
1. Safe Flooring

- Slip-Resistant Surfaces: Use flooring materials that provide good traction, such as non-slip vinyl or rubber flooring. Avoid carpets with thick padding or loose rugs that can cause tripping hazards
- Level Surfaces: Ensure all walking surfaces are firm and even, minimizing the risk of unexpected changes in elevation

2. Adequate Lighting

- Bright and Even Lighting: Install bright, non-flickering lights throughout the home to improve visibility. This includes using energy-efficient bulbs and ensuring that light switches are easily accessible
- Nightlights and Motion Sensors: Place nightlights in hallways and bathrooms, and consider motion-sensor lights to illuminate paths during nighttime3. Clutter-Free Spaces

- Clear Walkways: Keep all pathways free from clutter, furniture, and obstacles to allow for safe navigation. Regularly assess areas for potential tripping hazards like loose items or uneven surfaces
- Organized Storage: Use storage solutions like bins and trays to keep items organized and out of sight, reducing visual clutter that can overwhelm individuals with vestibular disorders
- 4. Supportive Furniture

- Sturdy Seating: Choose chairs and beds that are easy to get in and out of, with armrests for added support. Avoid low furniture that may require bending down too far
- Grab Bars: Install grab bars in key areas such as bathrooms, near toilets, and in hallways to provide additional support when standing or moving
- 5. Bathroom Safety

- Non-Slip Mats: Use non-slip mats in the shower and around the toilet to prevent slips
- Raised Toilet Seats: Consider installing raised toilet seats to assist with sitting down and standing up more easily6. Emergency Preparedness

- Personal Alarm Systems: Implement a personal emergency response system (PERS) that allows individuals to alert others in case of a fall or emergency
- Accessible Exits: Ensure multiple exits from the home are clear and easy to navigate in case of emergencies
- 7. Health Management Resources

- **Regular Health Check-ups: Schedule** routine appointments with healthcare providers to monitor vertigo symptoms and adjust treatment as necessary
- **Vestibular Rehabilitation Therapy (VRT): Consider** engaging in VRT to improve balance and reduce dizziness through targeted exercises

8. Environmental Adjustments

Minimize Noise and Glare: Use soundproofing techniques if necessary, and reduce glare from

Chapter 9: Building a Support System

- The importance of emotional and social support in recovery.

The importance of **emotional and social support** in the recovery of vertigo patients cannot be overstated. Living with vertigo can be challenging, as it often leads to feelings of anxiety, frustration, and isolation. Here are several key aspects that highlight the significance of emotional and social support for individuals dealing with this condition:

1. Reduction of Anxiety and Stress

- **Emotional Well-being:** Vertigo can induce significant anxiety due to unpredictable episodes and the fear of falling. Emotional support from family, friends, or support groups can help alleviate these feelings, providing a sense of security and understanding

- **Coping Strategies:** Engaging with mental health professionals or support groups can equip patients with coping strategies to manage stress and anxiety effectively. Techniques such as meditation and deep breathing exercises can also be beneficial in reducing symptoms associated with vertigo

2. Enhanced Recovery Process

- **Motivation for Rehabilitation:** Emotional support encourages adherence to treatment plans, including vestibular rehabilitation therapy (VRT). A supportive environment can motivate patients to participate actively in exercises designed to improve balance and reduce dizziness

- **Shared Experiences:** Connecting with others who have similar experiences can provide valuable insights and encouragement, making the recovery process feel less isolating. Sharing stories within support groups can foster hope and resilience
- 3. **Improved Communication**

- **Understanding Symptoms:** Open communication with loved ones about the challenges faced due to vertigo can lead to better understanding and adjustments in daily activities. This can help create a more accommodating environment that reduces triggers for vertigo episodes
- **Advocacy:** Emotional support networks can also assist patients in advocating for their needs within healthcare settings, ensuring they receive appropriate care and resources.

4. **Social Engagement**

- **Combating Isolation:** Social support helps combat feelings of isolation that may arise from avoiding activities due to fear of vertigo episodes. Encouragement from friends and family to engage in social activities can enhance quality of life
- **Community Resources:** Accessing community resources, such as local support groups or online forums, provides additional avenues for social interaction and shared learning about managing vertigo.

5. **Holistic Health Approach**

- **Integrative Health Services:** Many healthcare providers offer integrative health services that focus on both physical and emotional well-being. This includes practices like acupuncture or mindfulness meditation, which can help relax the body and alleviate tension related to vertigo symptoms

- **Comprehensive Care:** Addressing both emotional and physical aspects of health leads to a more comprehensive approach to recovery, improving overall outcomes for patients with vertigo.

In conclusion, emotional and social support play a vital role in the recovery journey for individuals experiencing vertigo. By fostering a supportive environment that addresses both emotional well-being and practical needs, patients are more likely to navigate their condition effectively and improve their quality of life.

- Tips for communicating balance disorders to friends and family.

Communicating balance disorders to friends and family is essential for fostering understanding and support. Here are some effective tips to help convey your experiences and needs:

Tips for Communicating Balance Disorders

1. Educate Your Loved Ones

- **Explain the Condition:** Share information about your specific balance disorder, including symptoms, triggers, and how it affects your daily life. This can help them understand what you are experiencing.

- **Use Simple Language:** Avoid medical jargon when possible; instead, use relatable terms to describe your condition.

2. Share Personal Experiences

- **Describe Symptoms:** Explain how balance issues manifest for you, such as feelings of dizziness, unsteadiness, or spatial disorientation. Sharing personal anecdotes can make your experiences more relatable.
- **Discuss Triggers:** Inform them about specific situations or environments that exacerbate your symptoms, so they can be more mindful in those contexts.

3. Express Your Needs

- **Be Clear About Support:** Let them know how they can help you—whether it's offering assistance during outings, helping with household tasks, or simply being patient during conversations.
- **Set Boundaries:** If certain activities or environments are challenging, communicate these boundaries clearly to avoid misunderstandings.

4. Encourage Open Dialogue

- **Invite Questions:** Encourage family and friends to ask questions if they're unsure about something. This promotes a better understanding of your condition.
- **Share Resources:** Provide articles or resources that explain balance disorders in more detail. This can help them grasp the complexities of your situation.

5. Discuss Emotional Impact

- **Talk About Feelings:** Share how living with a balance disorder affects your emotional well-being. Discuss any feelings of anxiety or frustration that may arise from your condition.
- **Highlight the Importance of Support:** Emphasize how emotional and social support can positively impact your recovery and daily life.

6. Use Visual Aids

- **Demonstrate Symptoms:** If comfortable, demonstrate what it feels like to experience dizziness or imbalance. This can create empathy and a better understanding of your challenges.
- **Visual Resources:** Consider using diagrams or videos that illustrate how balance works in the body and what happens when it is disrupted.

7. Keep Communication Ongoing

- **Regular Updates:** Keep family and friends informed about any changes in your condition or treatment plan. This helps them stay engaged and supportive.
- **Check In Frequently:** Encourage regular conversations about how you're feeling and any adjustments that might be needed in their support.

By effectively communicating about balance disorders, you can foster a supportive environment that enhances understanding and compassion from friends and family, ultimately aiding in your recovery process.

- Online and local support networks for individuals and caregivers.

For individuals and caregivers of vertigo patients, finding support through online and local networks can be invaluable. Here are some resources and options available:

Online Support Networks

1. Social Media Groups:

- **Facebook Groups:** Several groups provide a platform for sharing experiences and coping strategies. Notable groups include:
    - Vestibular Disorders Support Group
    - Vertigo Support Group
    - Dizzy and Vertigo Support Group

2. Online Forums:

- Platforms like Reddit host communities where individuals can discuss their experiences with vertigo, share advice, and find encouragement from others facing similar challenges

3. Dedicated Websites:

- **Vestibular Disorders Association (VEDA):** This organization offers resources, articles, and a directory of support groups that can be beneficial for both patients and caregivers. Their website is a great starting point for finding local chapters and support

4. Telehealth Services:

- Many healthcare providers now offer telehealth options for counseling and therapy related to vestibular disorders. This can be a convenient way to access professional support from home.

Local Support Networks
1. Community Health Centers:

- Many local health centers offer support groups specifically for individuals with balance disorders. These groups provide a safe space to share experiences and receive emotional support.

2. Rehabilitation Centers:

- Facilities like NYU Langone offer specialized programs that combine vestibular therapy with psychological support services, helping individuals manage both physical symptoms and emotional challenges

3. Local Chapters of National Organizations:

- Check for local chapters of organizations like VEDA or the American Academy of Otolaryngology-Head and Neck Surgery, which may host support groups or informational sessions.

4. Caregiver Support Groups:

- Many communities have caregiver support networks that focus on providing resources and emotional support to those caring for individuals with chronic conditions, including vertigo.

Additional Resources

- **Counseling Services:** Seek out therapists who specialize in vestibular disorders or chronic illness management. They can provide coping strategies for both patients and caregivers.

- **Educational Workshops:** Some hospitals and community centers offer workshops on managing vertigo, which can be beneficial for both patients and their families.
- **Podcasts and Blogs:** There are various podcasts and blogs dedicated to vestibular disorders that share personal stories, expert advice, and coping strategies.

By utilizing these online and local support networks, individuals with vertigo and their caregivers can find community, understanding, and practical resources to navigate the challenges associated with this condition.

- Encouragement to share experiences and learn from others.

Sharing experiences is a powerful tool for individuals dealing with balance disorders like vertigo, as it fosters connection, validation, and personal growth. Here are some key points highlighting the importance of sharing experiences and learning from others:

1. **Connection and Belonging**

- **Building Relationships:** Sharing personal stories creates opportunities for connection and fosters relationships based on mutual understanding. When individuals express their challenges and triumphs, it helps others feel less isolated, reinforcing the idea that they are not alone in their struggles
- **Empathy Development:** Engaging in conversations about shared experiences enhances empathy among participants. This mutual sharing allows individuals to step into each other's shoes, promoting a deeper understanding of one

another's feelings and situations

2. Validation of Feelings

- **Feeling Understood:** When individuals share their experiences, they often find that others relate to their struggles. This validation can be incredibly comforting, as it reassures them that their feelings are normal and shared by others facing similar challenges
- **Encouragement to Open Up:** The act of sharing encourages others to disclose their own experiences, creating a supportive environment where vulnerability is welcomed and appreciated

3. Learning and Growth

- **Gaining Insights:** Sharing experiences allows individuals to learn from one another's journeys. Hearing how others have navigated similar challenges can provide practical advice and new coping strategies that may be beneficial in managing their own conditions
- **Resilience Building:** Discussing both positive and negative experiences can enhance resilience. Individuals can reflect on how they overcame obstacles, which can inspire hope and motivate others in their recovery journeys

4. Emotional Recovery

- **Facilitating Healing:** Sharing stories can promote emotional recovery by encouraging individuals to process their feelings and experiences. This communal aspect of healing helps reduce feelings of loneliness and depression often associated with chronic conditions like vertigo

- **Creating a Supportive Community:** Engaging with support groups or online forums where individuals share their journeys fosters a sense of community. This environment provides reassurance that others understand what they are going through, which can be immensely comforting

5. Encouragement for Others

- **Inspiring Hope:** Hearing success stories from others who have managed their balance disorders can instill hope in those currently struggling. These narratives serve as reminders that improvement is possible, motivating individuals to continue seeking help and exploring treatment options
- **Empowering Others:** By sharing their own experiences, individuals empower others to take control of their situations, encouraging proactive approaches to managing symptoms.

In conclusion, sharing experiences is vital for individuals with balance disorders like vertigo. It promotes connection, validation, learning, emotional recovery, and inspiration among peers. Encouraging open dialogue about these experiences not only benefits the individual sharing but also enriches the community as a whole, fostering a supportive network for all involved.

- **windows with sheer blinds or curtains to create a more comfortable environment**
- **Simplified Décor: Opt for simple patterns and neutral colors in furnishings to avoid overwhelming visual stimuli**

that can trigger symptoms

By incorporating these components into the home environment, individuals with vertigo can significantly enhance their safety, comfort, and overall quality of life.

chapter 10: Living with Balance Disorders

1. Real-life stories of individuals successfully managing balance disorders.

Individuals facing balance disorders often find themselves navigating a challenging path, but many have successfully managed their conditions through various methods, including physical therapy, lifestyle adjustments, and support systems. Here are some inspiring real-life stories of individuals who have triumphed over balance disorders:

Personal Success Stories

1. Overcoming BPPV

One individual shared their journey after experiencing balance issues following a whiplash injury. Initially struggling with daily activities, they sought physical therapy and learned specific exercises to manage their symptoms, particularly for Benign Paroxysmal Positional Vertigo (BPPV). By avoiding caffeine and incorporating B-vitamin supplements into their routine, they gradually regained confidence and mobility. After nearly nine years of managing their condition, they reported significant improvement and a return to normalcy in their life

2. Concussion Recovery

Another success story comes from a patient recovering from a concussion who faced persistent dizziness and headaches. Under the guidance of a physiotherapist, they engaged in vestibular rehabilitation that included tailored exercises to improve balance and coordination. Over time, the patient regained confidence and was able to resume activities such as swimming and running, demonstrating the effectiveness of targeted physical therapy in overcoming vestibular disorders

3. A Journey from Fear to Confidence

Lucia, a 65-year-old woman who developed a fear of falling after a minor home accident, sought help at a balance clinic. Through comprehensive assessments and personalized balance improvement techniques, she was able to conquer her fears and regain her independence. Her journey highlights how targeted interventions can significantly enhance quality of life for those with balance concerns

4. Managing Chronic Ear Issues

Jessica Nonamaker's battle with vertigo stemmed from chronic ear problems that led to significant quality-of-life issues. After receiving a series of therapeutic movements known as the Epley maneuver and engaging in regular physical therapy sessions, she experienced substantial relief from her symptoms. This coordinated care approach allowed her to reclaim her daily activities and enjoy family time without the debilitating effects of vertigo

5. Restoring Independence

Lenora M., who had been severely affected by vertigo, found hope through physical therapy that addressed her specific balance issues. After undergoing treatment that included repositioning maneuvers for BPPV, she regained her confidence and independence. Lenora's story emphasizes the importance of motivation and targeted rehabilitation in overcoming debilitating balance disorders

Key Takeaways

- **Physical Therapy**: Many individuals found success through tailored physical therapy programs that focused on specific exercises to improve balance.
- **Lifestyle Adjustments**: Dietary changes, such as avoiding caffeine or incorporating supplements like B-vitamins, played a crucial role in managing symptoms.
- **Support Systems**: The encouragement and expertise of healthcare professionals were vital in guiding patients through their recovery journeys.
- **Persistence**: Consistent effort in rehabilitation exercises led to significant improvements in daily functioning and overall quality of life.

These stories reflect the resilience of individuals dealing with balance disorders and the potential for recovery through appropriate treatment strategies. Each journey is unique but underscores the importance of seeking help and staying committed to rehabilitation efforts.

1. Long-term strategies for maintaining stability in everyday life.

Maintaining stability in everyday life, especially for individuals managing balance disorders or other health challenges, requires a proactive approach. Here are long-term strategies that can help ensure stability:

FINDING YOUR BALANCE , A GUIDE TO STABILITY IN LIFE

Long-Term Strategies for Maintaining Stability

1. Establish a Routine

- **Consistency**: Develop a daily routine that includes regular times for meals, exercise, and rest. This structure can help manage symptoms and create a sense of normalcy.
- **Sleep Hygiene**: Prioritize good sleep habits to improve overall well-being and cognitive function.

2. Physical Activity

- **Tailored Exercise Programs**: Engage in physical therapy or specific exercises designed to improve balance and coordination. Activities like tai chi or yoga can enhance stability and flexibility.
- **Regular Movement**: Incorporate light physical activity into daily routines, such as walking or stretching, to promote circulation and reduce stiffness.

3. Nutrition and Hydration

- **Balanced Diet**: Focus on a nutritious diet rich in fruits, vegetables, whole grains, and lean proteins to support overall health.
- **Stay Hydrated**: Ensure adequate fluid intake, as dehydration can exacerbate balance issues.

4. Environmental Adaptations

- **Home Modifications**: Make necessary adjustments at home, such as removing tripping hazards, using non-slip mats, and installing grab bars in bathrooms.

- **Assistive Devices**: Consider using mobility aids like canes or walkers if necessary to enhance safety while moving.

5. Mental Health Support

- **Mindfulness and Relaxation Techniques**: Practice mindfulness, meditation, or breathing exercises to reduce anxiety and improve focus.
- **Counseling or Support Groups**: Engage with mental health professionals or support groups to share experiences and coping strategies.

6. Continuous Learning and Adaptation

- **Stay Informed**: Keep up with the latest research on balance disorders and management techniques to adapt strategies as needed.
- **Skill Development**: Participate in workshops or courses that focus on balance training or related skills.

7. Social Connections

- **Build a Support Network**: Maintain strong relationships with family and friends who can provide emotional support and practical assistance.
- **Community Engagement**: Join local groups or classes that focus on activities promoting balance and social interaction.

8. Regular Monitoring

- **Health Check-ups**: Schedule regular appointments with healthcare providers to monitor progress and adjust treatment plans as necessary.
- **Self-Assessment**: Keep track of symptoms and triggers to identify patterns that may require intervention.

By implementing these strategies, individuals can foster a stable environment that supports their health needs while enhancing their quality of life. Each strategy contributes to building resilience against the challenges posed by balance disorders or other health conditions.

1. Encouraging a positive outlook and resilience in the face of challenges.

Encouraging a positive outlook and resilience in the face of challenges is essential for personal growth and well-being. Here are effective strategies to foster this mindset:

Strategies for Encouraging a Positive Outlook and Resilience

1. Cultivate Strong Relationships

- **Connect with Others**: Building and maintaining relationships with friends and family can provide emotional support during tough times. Engaging in open conversations can ease stress and foster a sense of belonging
- **Seek Support**: Don't hesitate to reach out for help from mentors or support groups. Sharing experiences can provide new perspectives and coping strategies

2. Practice Gratitude

- **Acknowledge Positives**: Regularly reflecting on what you are grateful for, even small things, can shift your focus from negative to positive aspects of life. This practice can improve mood and overall outlook

Gratitude Journaling: Keeping a journal to note daily gratitudes can reinforce this habit and serve as a reminder during challenging times.

3. Maintain a Hopeful Perspective

- **Visualize Success**: Instead of dwelling on fears or problems, visualize positive outcomes and what you want to achieve. This forward-thinking approach can motivate you to take constructive actions
- **Focus on Solutions**: Train yourself to look for solutions rather than fixating on problems. This shift in mindset fosters resilience and encourages proactive behavior

4. Engage in Self-Care

- **Physical Activity**: Regular exercise has been shown to reduce stress, anxiety, and depression while boosting mood. Activities like yoga or walking can enhance both physical and mental health.
- **Mindfulness Practices**: Techniques such as meditation or deep breathing can help manage stress levels and promote a sense of calm amid challenges.

5. Learn from Setbacks

- **Reflect on Experiences**: Analyze past challenges to identify lessons learned. Understanding what went wrong can help you develop better strategies for the future

- **Embrace Change**: Recognize that change is a part of life. Adapting to new circumstances can strengthen your resilience over time.

6. Set Realistic Goals

- **Break Down Challenges**: Set achievable goals that allow you to make incremental progress. Celebrating small victories can boost confidence and motivation.
- **Stay Flexible**: Be open to adjusting your goals as circumstances change, which allows you to remain resilient in the face of unexpected challenges.

7. Engage in Helping Others

- **Volunteer Work**: Helping others can provide a sense of purpose and control, enhancing your own well-being while fostering connections with your community
- **Acts of Kindness**: Simple acts of kindness can improve your mood and create positive interactions that reinforce social bonds.

8. Seek Professional Guidance

- **Therapy or Counseling**: Professional support can provide valuable tools for managing stress and building resilience. Therapists can help you develop coping strategies tailored to your unique situation

By integrating these strategies into daily life, individuals can cultivate a more positive outlook and enhance their resilience in the face of life's inevitable challenges. Each step taken towards fostering these qualities contributes significantly to overall mental health and well-being.

Suggestions for ongoing learning and self-advocacy in health management

Ongoing learning and self-advocacy are crucial components of effective health management. They empower individuals to take charge of their health, make informed decisions, and engage actively with healthcare providers. Here are some suggestions to foster these qualities:

Suggestions for Ongoing Learning in Health Management

1. **Stay Informed**

- **Read Medical Literature**: Regularly review journals, articles, and reputable online resources to keep up with the latest research and treatment options relevant to your health condition
- **Utilize Technology**: Leverage apps and online platforms that provide updates on health trends, medication information, and wellness tips.

2. **Engage in Continuous Education**

- **Attend Workshops and Seminars**: Participate in local or online workshops that focus on health management topics relevant to your needs. This can include nutrition, exercise, or specific medical conditions
- **Enroll in Courses**: Consider taking courses on health literacy or self-management strategies through community colleges or online platforms.

3. **Network with Peers**

- **Join Support Groups**: Engage with others who share similar health challenges. Support groups can provide valuable insights and shared experiences that enhance understanding and coping strategies.
- **Participate in Community Health Events**: These events often feature speakers and resources that can deepen your knowledge about managing health conditions.

Suggestions for Self-Advocacy in Health Management
1. **Communicate Effectively with Healthcare Providers**

- **Prepare for Appointments**: Write down questions or concerns before visits to ensure you cover all important topics during consultations. Bring a list of medications and symptoms to discuss
- **Be Honest About Your Health**: Share all relevant information with your healthcare provider, including lifestyle factors and any changes in symptoms.

2. **Understand Your Rights**

- **Know Your Patient Rights**: Familiarize yourself with your rights as a patient, including the right to receive clear information about your diagnosis, treatment options, and the right to participate in decision-making regarding your care
- **Request Second Opinions**: If uncertain about a diagnosis or treatment plan, don't hesitate to seek a second opinion from another qualified healthcare professional.

3. **Develop a Personal Health Plan**

- **Set Clear Goals**: Work with your healthcare provider to establish realistic health goals tailored to your needs. This can include lifestyle changes, medication adherence, or therapy participation.
- **Monitor Your Progress**: Keep track of your health metrics (e.g., blood pressure, weight) and symptoms over time. This data can help you advocate for necessary adjustments in your care plan.

4. Utilize Available Resources

- **Access Patient Advocacy Organizations**: Many organizations offer resources for patients seeking information on specific conditions, treatments, and rights.
- **Leverage Online Forums**: Engage in online communities where you can ask questions and share experiences related to health management.

By integrating these strategies into daily life, individuals can cultivate a proactive approach to their health management through ongoing learning and self-advocacy. This empowerment not only enhances personal well-being but also fosters better communication and collaboration with healthcare providers.

About the Author

Head of the Department of ENT, Jubilee Mission Medical College , South India